Cognitive Behavioral Therapy:

Retrain Your Brain to Overcome Depression, Anxiety, and Panic Attacks with CBT.

12 Easy Strategies Made to Find Happiness and Freedom

Written By: George B. Wells

© Copyright George B. Wells 2019

All rights reserved.

The content contained within this book may not be reproduced, duplicated or transmitted without direct written permission from the author or the publisher.

Under no circumstances will any blame or legal responsibility be held against the publisher, or author, for any damages, reparation, or monetary loss due to the information contained within this book, either directly or indirectly.

Legal Notice:
This book is copyright protected. It is only for personal use. You cannot amend, distribute, sell, use, quote or paraphrase any part, or the content within this book, without the consent of the author or publisher.

Disclaimer Notice:
Please note the information contained within this document is for educational and entertainment purposes only. All effort has been executed to present accurate, up to date, reliable, complete information. No warranties of any kind are declared or implied. Readers acknowledge that the author is not engaging in the rendering of legal, financial, medical or professional advice. The content within this book has been derived from various sources. Please consult a licensed professional before attempting any techniques outlined in this book.

By reading this document, the reader agrees that under no circumstances is the author responsible for any losses, direct or indirect, that are incurred as a result of the use of information contained within this document, including, but not limited to, errors, omissions, or inaccuracies.

Contents Page

Introduction 7
Chapter 1 - Cognitive Behavioral Therapy (CBT) 12
    What is Cognitive Behavioral Therapy (CBT)? 12
    The History of CBT 13
    Understanding CBT 19
    What is CBT for? 20
    How can CBT help me and why? 21
    Why is CBT an Effective Therapy? 22
Chapter 2 - The Basics of CBT 24
    What is the CBT Process? 24
    What are the Basic Principles of CBT treatment? .. 26
    What are automatic thoughts? 27
    What are intrusive thoughts? 28
    Automatic Thought Patterns 28
    Our Rules and Assumptions 29
Chapter 3 - Applications for CBT 31
    Anxiety and Panic Attacks 31
    Phobias, Post Traumatic Stress Disorder (PTSD), and Obsessive-Compulsive Disorder (OCD) 34
    Depression 36
    Anger Management 38
    Is CBT an Effective Treatment for Children and Adolescents? 39
Chapter 4 – What's my Problem? 42
    Strategy 1 – Identifying your irrational and negative thinking patterns and actions with Journaling. 43

What are Cognitive Distortions? 45
Defining Cognitive Distortions 45
Strategy 2 – Identifying and Making Sense of
Cognitive Distortions 51
Chapter 5 – Going Deeper into your Problems 55
Strategy 3 – Identifying, Assessing and
Challenging Bodily Reactions 55
Strategy 4 - Assessing Problem Causes Using
the ABC Model 61
Defining Problems 65
Chapter 6 - Identify and Challenge your Core Beliefs 68
Mistakes 68
Strategy 5 - Self-Acceptance 70
Core Beliefs 72
Facing Problems, Assumptions and Beliefs
Head-on 76
Strategy 6 - Exposure Planning 77
Understanding your Assumptions and Beliefs 79
Strategy 7 Directly Targeting your Negative Core
Beliefs 81
Chapter 7 – Relax, Regroup, and Believe 85
Strategy 8 – Relaxed breathing techniques 85
Move Beliefs from your Intellect to your Essence .. 89
Negativity versus Creativity 90
Strategy 9 - Muscle relaxation 91
Turn your Negativity into Creativity 93
Chapter 8 – Goal Setting for Greater Good 97
Problem Focused and Goal Orientated 97
Strategy 10 – Positive Prediction Planning 99
Strategy 11 - Finding your Focus 101

How to set Effective Goals 104
Top 3 Tips for Goal Setting 106
Strategy 12 - Targeting your Triggers 109
Chapter 9 – Other CBT Techniques 113
Assertiveness in CBT 113
Five Top Tips to increase your Assertiveness 115
Awareness Training 117
Chapter 10 – Mindfulness-Based Cognitive Therapy (MBCT) 122
Mindfulness Based Cognitive Therapy Versus Cognitive Behavioral Therapy 122
Important ideas in Mindfulness-based Cognitive Therapy 124
How does MBCT Work? 124
Problems that may be addressed by MBCT 125
MBCT Techniques and Exercises 126
Benefits of Mindfulness 129
Mindfulness Skills 129
Other Alternative Cognitive Behavioral Approaches 130
Chapter 11 - CBT Treatment 133
How will I know if CBT is for me? 133
Do I need a Therapist? 135
What Should I Expect on my First Visit with a CBT Therapist? 136
What Happens in a CBT Session? 137
How Long does CBT Last and How Frequent are the Sessions? 139
How do I Find the Right CBT Therapist for me? .. 139
Why do I Need to have a Good, Collaborative, Therapeutic Relationship with my Therapist? 141

Will the CBT Therapist be able to Understand
　　and Appreciate my own Background? 142
　　What about medications? 144
Chapter 12 – Maintenance.. 145
　　How to Maintain Automatic Thoughts and
　　Cognitive Distortions... 146
　　Find the Full and Objective Perspective 147
　　Emotional Reasoning 148
　　Forging New Synapses 148
　　Avoiding Backsliding... 148
　　Keep up CBT 149
　　How your New Healthy Brain Functions 150
Chapter 13 – BONUS CHAPTER: Ten Ways that CBT Techniques can be Used to Boost your Energy... 152
Conclusion 159
The Cognitive Behavioral Therapy Workbook ... 161
　　Reference List 210

Introduction

"There are three musts that hold us back: I must do well. You must treat me well. And the world must be easy.
Ellis, A. (Brainyquote.com, 2019) [1]*"*

Life can be hectic and busy. It's not always easy to relax or take a moment to ourselves when we constantly live, work and breathe in pressurized environments. On a daily basis we deal with situations that affect us both mentally and physically so it's natural for us to feel overwhelmed as a result. Sometimes we want to escape but we can't exactly escape our mind, *so what can we do?*

The mind is complex as we don't always control our thoughts and how we feel. Stress is common, in fact it's probably more common than you think. It's everywhere and it deprives us of life's little pleasures because if we're stressed, it's hard to enjoy anything. Self-care can help us to lower our stress levels, but this is something that we barely make time for. *Sound familiar?*

We've all been there! Yet, self-care is often underrated. It's so important because the strain can become too much and this can lead to anxiety, depression, panic attacks, and intrusive thoughts as all the negativity we feel bears weight on our shoulders. The most important thing we can do in this situation is to acknowledge the struggles we face and that's not always easy. People often choose to ignore their problems, but ignorance is not bliss for long, because we can't ignore them forever. They build inside and increase with intensity, and this makes us miserable. Unhappiness can affect our mind and it slowly creeps out. The way we appear and behave starts to reflect this.

On occasion, we need a little help in order to work things out and improve our mental health. That's okay, people should always get help if they need it but again, we arrive at the very first step of dealing with a problem, and that's acknowledgement and acceptance. Once we acknowledge that we have a problem and accept that we need to do something about it, we can start considering solutions. We may need help from a therapist, especially in the beginning as this can really help us to identify what exactly it is that's affecting us. This isn't always a long-term solution as we may need to learn how to maintain our mental health. *Wouldn't it be great if we had the tools and skills we need to help and maintain our mental health?* Well you can! It's time to act and overcome these issues before they take hold and we can do this with Cognitive Behavioral Therapy.

If you want to make positive changes in your life because of how you feel, and you're not sure how, this book is for you. That means you've accepted that something must change in your life, and that's a positive step. If you're ready to review your feelings and behavior, address the problems in your life, and develop strategies and coping techniques that improve your state of mind then you've come to the right place.

Cognitive Behavioral Therapy (CBT) is designed to help you address the negative patterns in your life. It's a structured and systematic approach of looking at and dealing with pessimistic beliefs and behaviors that impact your life. CBT can have long-term benefits as it is an efficient, effective and long-lasting treatment for many psychological problems.

This book gives you a comprehensive introduction to CBT, but it will also help you to develop workable techniques that you can adopt into your life. It explores the different approaches and types of therapies on offer and will encourage you to question the assumptions you have on autopilot in relation to yourself and other people. CBT generally concentrates on the present but with knowledge and practice, it can also change the way you feel about your past and it can help you escape from the negative thinking patterns that haunt your mind. With your newly found freedom and flexibility, you will no longer be held back and can start looking forward to the future.

In order to become happier and improve your mindset, you must be open-minded when reading this book and willing to try the skills and methods suggested. You may find that you need a Cognitive Behavioral Therapist to help you identify and make the changes but if you are susceptible to the change, this simple shift in how we think and what we believe has so many benefits. Be careful not to confuse the word simple, with easy. CBT methods take time and practice, although it can be very enlightening.

CBT is a lifestyle change because it challenges the way you think, and thinking is an automatic brain function. It can give you back control and if you commit yourself you will reap the rewards. It's time to take charge of your own destiny, so now I ask you; *do you choose to stay stagnant, or will you embrace this possibly life-changing experience?*

Cognitive Behavioral Therapy is not a magic formula, but more a way of life that you can adopt into your routine to help you to rationalize and make sense of your thoughts and feelings, before they get out of control. In chapter 1, you will get your first taste of CBT (if you're not already familiar) as we'll explore what CBT is, how it was developed and how it can help us. As we move through the chapters, we will discover the principles of CBT, why this type of therapy works, and we'll look at CBT in depth by exploring its core beliefs and how we can apply this to our own individual situation. Be prepared, as CBT will push you to a whole new level as we look at goal setting and problem solving, possible treatments and practice, before we look at to mindfulness practices.

This book aims to inspire you by giving you the whole picture and towards the end of this book, we cover one of the most important parts of CBT, maintenance. As mentioned earlier, this is a lifestyle change so it's important to nurture and maintain a healthy state of mind. If you want to find out how to do that, then you should certainly read this book.

Remember, CBT leads to a happy life!

Chapter 1 - Cognitive Behavioral Therapy (CBT)

So, what is cognitive behavioral therapy? If you're not already familiar with CBT, this question will certainly be in your mind right now. We already know that behavior is the way we act, and cognitive is to do with the mind, *but what do we really mean when we refer to Cognitive Behavioral Therapy?* You're about to find out because we're going to review this therapy and find out what it is exactly. We are going to go back to the roots of CBT, look at its history and discuss key theorists that developed CBT. This will help you to gain a stronger understanding of this topic, so we can find out how and why it can help you.

What is Cognitive Behavioral Therapy (CBT)?

Cognitive Behavioral Therapy is a kind of therapy that helps you alter your beliefs, as well as the way you behave and think. Mental health charity, Mind, suggests that this is a kind of talking treatment that teaches you important coping skills. They say that we can suffer negative emotions if we interpret a situation badly. They then suggest that we react and behave in a particular way because of this negative attitude (Mind, 2019).[2]

CBT in itself works to break this cycle. It helps you to change those negative thought patterns and focus on your current problems. It looks for ways to alter your state of mind every day, and this way it becomes part of your routine until you change your beliefs and attitudes. Of course, you have to work at this by using a range of CBT tools, skills and methods. CBT incorporates effective coping strategies that help with depression and anxiety related conditions, though it is not limited to these.

Dobson and Dozios (2010), claim that Cognitive Behavioral Therapies share three fundamental propositions at their core and they include the ideas that "cognitive activity affects behavior, cognitive activity may be monitored and altered, and desired behavior change may be effected through cognitive change."(Dobson, 2010, p.4.)[3]

Throughout this chapter, we are going to find out more about CBT, so that you have a stronger understanding of this. We will think about what it is and how it can help us.

The History of CBT

Cognitive Behavioral Therapy has been practiced much longer than most people probably think, as over the last few years this has increased its popularity and become better known. As CBT is both cognitive therapy and behavior therapy combined, it focuses on three key areas: how we think, feel and behave. *Simply Psychology* state that Cognitive Behavioral Therapy is "an umbrella term for many different therapies that share some common elements" and that's very true. The therapy itself can treat a wide variety of problems because it works on those three key areas, and ensures improvements are made across the board. Although Cognitive Behavioral Therapy itself was practiced in the mid 1950's and early 1960's, it began much earlier as psychologists and psychotherapists developed and theorized their practices over this period (McLeod, 2019).[4]

One of the earliest therapies in CBT was Rational Emotive Behavior Therapy (REBT), and this was developed in the 1950's by psychotherapist, Albert Ellis. He was the first to confirm that in order to help a person be happy with others, they have to be happy with themselves. After becoming increasingly unhappy with the psychoanalytic approach. He then began experimenting and researching Greek and Roman Stoic philosophers and their work. These Ancient philosophers suggested that most people are not troubled by things, as it is actually their own beliefs and attitudes towards those things that causes the issue (Ellis and Dryden, 1997).[5] This idea formed the basis for REBT and is essentially how this therapy was born.

Rational Emotive Behavior Therapy focuses on emotional and behavioral problems. The therapy aims to help a person address their unreasonable beliefs and transform them, so that they become reasonable. The first step to REBT is identifying the beliefs that hold a person back and then it encourages them to challenge these ineffective and often untrue beliefs by reflecting and testing reality (McLeod, 2019).[6]

Albert Ellis's REBT theory concentrated on something he called **common irrational assumptions** and basically, they are referencing the ideas we hold in relation to ourselves.

According to McLeod (2019), in *Simply Psychology,* they are:
1. They believe that they should be competent at everything.
2. When things don't go their way, they view it as being a catastrophic event.
3. They feel that they have no control over their feelings or happiness.
4. They feel that they need someone to depend on and that person should be stronger than them.
5. They are defined by their past history and this influences their life right now.
6. They consider it disastrous if they can't find the perfect solution to their problem because they believe that perfect solutions exist. [7]

Ellis believes that if we can change these assumptions by altering our thinking patterns by following something that he called *The ABC Model*. This 3-column model is still used today to assess the changes that need to be made in beliefs, attitudes and thinking patterns and we discuss this in chapter 5.

Another instrumental figure in CBT is Aaron Beck. Beck is responsible for developing Cognitive Therapy in the late 1960's. His approach was more commonly used as therapy for depression and the therapist's aim is to help clients recognize how their negative thoughts can be destructive and can ultimately be responsible for their depressive state. According to *Simply Psychology,* Beck believed "That a person's reaction to specific upsetting thoughts may contribute to abnormality." (McLeod, 2019). He goes onto discuss how confronting our issues is often upsetting but it can also be comforting. Beck calls these "automatic thoughts" and again, this is down to think patterns, and how a person's negativity can cause depression. Therapists who use this method, often challenge these thoughts by getting their client to apply different ways of thinking or interpreting their thoughts and feelings.[8] Beck (1967), highlighted three mechanisms that he considers to be the main causes of depression. He developed the cognitive triad which demonstrates the negative views we have of ourselves, the world and future. Beck also thought that negative self-schemas, often developed in childhood, usually follow a traumatic event. They develop a negative attitude and are often very cynical as a result. The third cause of depression is a result of errors in logic. He calls these 'Cognitive Distortions' and considers them to be a form of illogical thinking. We talk in depth about cognitive distortions in chapter 4. Negative thought patterns and attitudes often leave people feeling defeated. This can ultimately lead to feelings of anxiety, stress and depression. It can also start off panic and feelings of anxiety.[9]

Again, Beck's aim was to change these thinking patterns and help people stray from negative thinking, by taking a different view or approach. His method of therapy focused on the client finding their own solution, through guidance from their therapist. It's only when we consider cognitive therapy and REBT together, that we can really start to understand CBT. Combining the two therapies certainly made sense and has proved effective over the years.

Behavioral Therapy roots go back to the early 1900's when papers were produced by Skinner, Pavlov and Watson. It wasn't until the 1940's when this type of therapy became popular mental disorders, due to the effects of war. Alfred Adler's focus on how basic mistakes being the cause of negative emotions in the early 1900's, inspired Albert Ellis's REBT. Adler is said to be one of the earliest psychotherapists to recognize cognition as a part of psychotherapy (Klear Minds, 2015)[10].

Cognitive Therapy and REBT combined started off the Cognitive Behavioral Therapy movement in the 1950's and 1960's yet no texts existed until the 1970s. Dobson (2010, p.4.) reflects on the work of Mahoney, who had claimed to have "undergone a 'cognitive revolution' in the 1960's" but following that, the focus continued on clinical psychology when considering theories. There were a number of models created for CBT but over time, they were developed.[11]

The combination of the two made sense because behavioral therapies like REBT, often addressed neurotic conditions that influenced behavior but did not conquer depression. Cognitive therapies involve talking. They are client-led and involve a certain amount of self-discovery or realization that includes identifying those unhelpful beliefs, then challenging them and modifying our behavior and thinking patterns. On the other hand, REBT is very confrontational as the therapist can point out the problems. The methods used in REBT often depend on the person as an individual, but the methods chosen in cognitive therapy are often focused on the specific condition.[12]

Understanding CBT

We have discussed the roots of CBT so by now, you should be gaining an understanding of Cognitive Behavioral Therapy. We have also discussed Cognitive Therapy and Behavioral Therapy as separate and merged entities, but in order to understand CBT, it is important to start with a good definition. Once we understand the basic concepts that form this therapy, the more likely we are to understand the mechanics and then, we can build on this to build a more in depth understanding.

Klear Minds (2015) give an excellent explanation of CBT:

CBT explores the relationship between feelings, thoughts, and behaviours. As such, it arose from two very distinct schools of psychology: behaviourism and cognitive therapy. It's roots can be traced in these two models and their subsequent merging. (Klear Minds, 2015)

It's obvious that CBT looks at the way we think, feel and behave because they are all linked together and disturbance in one, can influence another. For example, we are upset or angry, this will impact how we think and how we act. By using CBT approaches, all aspects are covered, and this is why this therapy is so successful. Merging cognitive and behavioral therapies was the real breakthrough in Cognitive Behavioral Therapy. As we move on to the different chapters in this book, we can start to enhance our understanding by exploring the different approaches and applying them. We now have a better understanding of CBT, so we can start to think about what it is actively used for.

What is CBT for?

CBT is used across the world to treat many health issues. In America, there are many private CBT professionals, and some counsellors and psychotherapists specialize in this as it's known to be an effective treatment method, especially for anxiety disorders and depression. Many people have a CBT therapist to help them and doctors are usually happy to refer on private clients for such therapy to help their patient, often before medication is prescribed, or to work alongside them. In the United Kingdom, it is actually promoted by the National Health Service (NHS) and they suggest that it is an effective and efficient way of treating many different mental health conditions. This includes depression, anxiety disorders, bipolar disorders, psychosis, borderline personality disorders, sleep problems and insomnia, panic disorders, anorexia, bulimia, phobias, obsessive consultant disorder, phobias, post-traumatic stress disorder, and also problems that relate to substance misuse. They also sometimes recommend CBT as a form of treatment for long-term health conditions like fibromyalgia, irritable bowel syndrome, and chronic fatigue syndrome. Obviously, this is not to suggest that CBT is always suitable for such conditions, but it has been known to help sufferers cope better with their symptoms (NHS UK, 2019).[13] CBT is now a recognized, well-researched and popular treatment, all over the world.

This list is not limited solely to these illnesses either, as on occasion, the treatment could be recommended for some other reason. Regardless, of what you use CBT for, there are certainly benefits for everyone. It can generally help you adopt a healthy mindset and become more mindful in your approaches to life.

How can CBT help me and why?

CBT can help you by challenging any beliefs, ideas, thinking patterns and behaviors that trouble you and cause difficulties. It helps you adopt a more open approach in which you can be honest with yourself. Sometimes in life we just have to let out how we feel and as this kind of therapy is recognized as a talking therapy, you can certainly do that.

With CBT you can work with a therapist or by yourself to identify these and then you focus on methods to change you in the future. It helps you to think in a more rational way and this can help you to alter the way you feel. CBT focuses on what's going on right now, but sometimes you can review your past and think about how the past has influenced the way you think and behave. It is not a quick fix, but you will discover new approaches, and use different methods that enable you to stop the cycle of negative thinking and behavior. Even if you sometimes revert to feeling to your old patterns, you will be able to stop and take a moment to reflect due to your newly found awareness. You will have the tools, skills and strategies you need to cope with your feelings and thoughts, which will ultimately alter your behavior (Mind, 2019)[14].

Why is CBT an Effective Therapy?

CBT is an effective therapy because of its personalized approach. It is problem-focused and goal-oriented when it comes to finding a solution, and it encourages you to learn proven strategies and skills to overcome and cope with problems in the long-term.

Think of CBT techniques as being your toolkit. You are given a range of tools to fix something, and it's up to you which one you choose. If it doesn't work, you can choose another. Cognitive Behavioral Therapy can help with many different problems because it addresses three things: thoughts, emotions and actions. These three things often work hand in hand because if we think of something, it can cause us to feel a specific way and act a specific way. CBT gets to the bottom of the whole problem because it's an all-rounded approach that attempts to change the way you think, assess your emotions and consider how you act, before you actually do anything automatically. It's a life skill that can help you lead a happy, positive and rational life.

Chapter 2 - The Basics of CBT

If you've made it to chapter 2, you must think that CBT sounds amazing and you're right but in order to start treatment, you need to know the basics. We all have to start somewhere, so don't worry if you are still getting to grips with CBT. Bobby Davro once said, "The measure of success is happiness and peace of mind." (Davro, 2019)[15] but happiness and peace of mind can also lead to your success as it's only with a clear mind, that we can start to truly seek out what we want in life.

It's time to explore the basics of CBT by discussing the CBT process, ideas and principles. Once we know what's causing our negative thoughts and behaviors, we can focus on CBT as a goal-orientated, problem-solving therapy. In order to understand Cognitive Behavioral Therapy and how we can use it, we first need to know the basic principles.

What is the CBT Process?

If you want to start with CBT, you need to know how it works. There is a very simple process, and the diagram below will help you understand how CBT can encourage you to identify and solve your problems.

You have a problem!
You might know you have a problem, but you might not be able to put your finger on what it is exactly. You turn to CBT to figure this out or solve it.

Identify your Problem
CBT will then encourage you to figure out what your problems are exactly and analyze those.

Set your Goals
Goal setting is an important part of CBT. Once you know your problems you can start to set goals by considering what your problems are right now, and what your ideal is. *What do you want?*

Problem Solving Time
Now you know what your problems are, it's time to dig deeper. Sure, CBT focuses on the now, but you need to work on your core beliefs, so that you can work on long-term change.

Apply the Techniques
When you're at the stage, you are really trying to make a difference. You're addressing your problems, aiming for your goals and changing your whole mindset. Keep trying and applying CBT until you achieve your goals.

Practice and Maintenance
It's important to build CBT methods into your daily life so that they become normal. There are several CBT techniques to try to build on, and you should maintain CBT to ensure you don't fall into repeating thought and behavior patterns.

What are the Basic Principles of CBT treatment?

We have discussed what CBT is already, but what are the basic principles? Well, in order to understand this, we need to think about the different concepts. Cognitive Behavioral Therapy is a type of psychotherapy that helps you change your automatic thought patterns, cope with your emotions, and challenge your negative behaviors. *Has anyone ever told you that your actions have consequences?* Well, they do! The way we react can stop us from moving on our lives, and that is why it is so important.

The basic principles of Cognitive Behavioral Therapy, lies within its name:
Cognitive = This is because the whole idea of CBT focuses on our ideas, beliefs, thoughts and generally how we feel.

Behavioral = You already know that behavior is something we do, or the way we act. Sometimes this can be driven by how we feel or our emotions.

Therapy = If we are in therapy, we are receiving treatment for something we have, are trying to work out, or fix it. The therapy eventually remedies the problem.

Think about an occasion when you've been reactionary. Maybe this is because someone takes something for you or treats you badly. We can be reactionary as our thoughts or behaviors are automatic, and as a result as we struggle to control our gut-reaction. This means we can't always help the way we feel or act, so we get emotional and behave without thinking. This is because we are programmed to think or react in a negative way instantly.

These basic principles indicate how this therapy is focused on what you think and how you act in relation to an event or trauma. They are like a gut-reaction as we respond without thinking. Our thoughts and behaviors occur regularly, *but what are automatic or intrusive thoughts and how can we change them?*

What are automatic thoughts?

Automatic thoughts are something that are triggered by a particular event or feeling, that stirs up a negative action, thought or behavior. It causes a reaction in one way or another and this can lead to feelings of anxiety, anger or depression. The word automatic has strong meaning here because if something is automatic, it is robotic, and it happens without thinking as it is an instant reaction. If you think of a machine doing something over and over again, that's how our brain works.

What are intrusive thoughts?

Intrusive thoughts are similar to automatic thoughts, but this is when you get distressed or disturbed by unwanted thoughts or images. Because of these thoughts, you are often triggered to act in a particular way, and you do compulsive things to help you cope with those thoughts. Intrusive thoughts are often intense, but they too happen automatically. Automatic thoughts are often negative thoughts that become a habit, but with intrusive thoughts, we don't want them to occur because of the way they make us feel and act.

Automatic Thought Patterns

Automatic thought patterns are commonly known in the CBT world as Cognitive Distortions. Grohl (2016) suggests that there are 15, but in this book, we have formed ten based on his studies (Ackerman, 2019).[16]

1. Filtering
2. Polarized thinking
3. Overgeneralization
4. Jumping to conclusions
5. Magnification or Minimization
6. Personalization
7. Blaming others
8. Dwell on what we should have done
9. False beliefs
10. Assuming we are always right

Cognitive distortions are categories that help us make sense of our automatic thoughts. The above distortions contribute to the assumptions, problems and beliefs we have in life. We discuss these cognitive distortions in detail in chapter 4. Be sure to check that out.

Cognitive distortions are a habit because our mind gets used to reacting in these negative patterns. Because they are automatic it can be tricky to see how we should react, because we react first and think later. Cognitive Behavioral Therapy is great at helping you to recognize these patterns and challenge or change them. As human beings we learn things all the time, so programming our mind to think or react differently is possible. We just have to learn it and limit ourselves in the same way we limit ourselves to treats when we are on a diet.

Our Rules and Assumptions

There are rules and assumptions we live by that can hold us back and this is exactly why CBT methods are useful because they challenge everything we live by, everything we believe in.

The way you think is something that is programmed into us. For example, sometimes people believe that if they come from a family that has struggled with their finances, they assume that they will always struggle too. In hindsight, it is scary to think that we do not believe that we can do better. Just because we've never had something, doesn't mean we never will.

It's also worth remembering that just because we have always had something, it doesn't mean we can't lose it. Being too complacent can also be a negative way of thinking, because we have to be rational. In contrast to the previous example, someone with money might believe that they can never lose it and that's not always the case. In order to be financially stable, we need to be smart with our money and have strategies or back-up plans in place. Changing all the rules and assumptions you live by that are negative or cause you anguish is at the heart of CBT and it can mean a happier and healthier you!

This chapter has covered the basics around Cognitive Behavioral Therapy, as well as different key techniques to consider, if you want to utilize this type of therapy and make changes in your life. In the next chapter. Now that we know the basics, it's important to learn about the different applications for CBT so that you can start to make a difference in your own life.

Chapter 3 - Applications for CBT

Have you ever felt down? Not quite good enough? Or so anxious that your functionality as a human being is affected? You're not on your own, most people have felt like this.

CBT can be used as a form of therapy for many different things, so we're going to focus on different ways to apply CBT techniques, based on your diagnosis. If you have medical diagnosis already, then you could have a head start. With CBT, treatments focus around both the person and the problem, so this is a great chapter to help you understand the techniques further.

Anxiety and Panic Attacks

You should have heard the word anxious or anxiety on quite a few occasions throughout this book already because CBT is a common treatment for anxiety.

But what exactly is anxiety?

Anxiety is that feeling of apprehension and dread that comes with the physical perception that something

> *bad might happen. It is accompanied by physical symptoms, such as increases in our heartbeat, breathing rate and muscle tension; tightness in the chest and sweating. (Edelman, 2006)*[17]

Anxiety is worry, but it's taken to a whole new level. It happens because we feel that something is about to happen, something that we don't like or want. We all feel anxious now and then, but this is often short-lived. Feeling anxious now and then is perfectly normal. It's that feeling you might get when you're going for that job interview and your heart races before you're called in. After a while, the feeling passes, and you continue with your day as normal.

Anxiety issues are disorders that are much more complex as they disturb our lives. The difference between the two is that anxiety issues or disorders mean that you might be so nervous and anxious that you never actually make the interview. They prevent you from even going. In fact, you may not have even applied for the job in the first place because the very thought of it is so overwhelming. CBT can really help with this.

We feel anxious when we feel that something threatens us. In the case of the job interview, we are threatened by our pride and ego, as we don't want to fail. Afterall, we are competing for a job that we may never get. Threats could be physical, mental, material, psychological, safety or even threats to our confidence and self-esteem. In turn, this influences the way we think and behave.

Severe anxiousness and worry can lead to panic attacks; when we are so worried and anxious that our mind and body start to react in various different ways that we can't control. Some people get chest pains, or their heart races, they can't hear or function properly, and they can even have blank moments and don't know how they got from one place to another. The panic hits an irrational level height that they can't escape from and it can be an awful, and sometimes terrifying experience. This is because we may not know what's going on around us and we become so frightened as we can't control our mind or bodily reactions.

Cognitive Behavioral Therapy is a useful form of therapy for anxiety and panic attacks because:
1. It helps you to explore and rationalize previous events that have created a sense of fear and make sense of them.
2. It helps you identify valuable coping techniques that work for you.
3. It encourages you to think differently and assess the worst-case scenario in a rational way, and the

probability of that actually happening.
4. It gives you focus and challenges you to achieve your progress goals.
5. It prepares and helps you face the situations that stir-up feelings of anxiousness.
6. Because its goal orientated, it keeps you motivated because you can monitor your progress.

Anxiety and panic attacks are something that need to be worked on over a long period of time, but CBT can really help to maintain focus and monitor progression. It can help you get to the bottom of your problems so that you understand the causes and triggers. This means you will have the tools you need to manage and cope with your anxiety and get on with your life before the panic sets in. Plus, if panic does start to creep up on you, you are able to recognize and cope with it before it gets out of control.

Phobias, Post Traumatic Stress Disorder (PTSD), and Obsessive-Compulsive Disorder (OCD)

Phobias, PTSD and OCD are all types of anxiety disorders. An important part of recovery when it comes to these types of anxiety issues is to accept them. These disorders are trickier to manage because they cause a physical reaction that can't be controlled.

Phobias - Anxiety is so intense when you have a phobia because you are consumed by fear. They are irrational and it often means that we blow situations out of proportion because we see them differently.

PTSD - A traumatic event is often the cause of PTSD and they can either be part of this event or simply witness it. The event stays with them, and they often suffer flashbacks of situations they have tried to block out or ignore. It's a high-state of anxiety that sets in feelings of fear and panic. Sometimes sufferers relive the traumatic event.

OCD - Anxiety is significantly elevated with this disorder because a person is often so consumed with rituals and struggle with change. This often stems from a fear that something bad is going to happen and the belief that the rituals will prevent it. People who suffer with OCD often have intrusive thoughts that haunt their mind. They feel a compulsion to prevent it and try to keep busy.

Cognitive Behavioral Therapy helps you to discover the cause of your anxiety disorders and face your fears. This can be traumatic for some people, so it's always important to get a formal diagnosis from a medical professional. CBT is known to be effective, but if the anxiety issues are severe, it's important to seek appropriate help and advice from a medical professional.

Depression

According to Markus MacGill (2017) in Medical News Today, *"Sadness, feeling down, having a loss of interest or pleasure in daily activities"* that persist and are left untreated can develop into depression. They explain that they can begin to hugely affect our life in a substantial way.[18] This definition is accurate because depression is such a broad condition that affects everyone in different ways. There are many scientific studies that express their support for CBT as a successful treatment for depression. This can often be successful with or without medication but remember, if you have been prescribed medication by a medical professional, you should never stop taking this, without professional medical advice.

When a person suffers from depression, they don't see the point of any change because of how they feel. They seem to adopt the negative attitude that nothing is ever going to change for them, and they struggle to see anything positive. People can suffer further symptoms that impact their energy levels; for example, they may lose their appetite or struggle to sleep and concentrate. All of these add to the misery-cloud that depression forms.

Typically, a negative event or experience causes depression, but negative core beliefs and assumptions can certainly build and result in this feeling too. Every person who suffers from depression will likely suffer from different triggers because the condition is individual, but the thoughts, feelings, and actions of a person who suffers from depression can be very similar.

CBT is an effective treatment for depression because:
1. It explores the root cause of your depression, which allows you to face your problems head-on, and focus on solving them.
2. It encourages you to stay focused by aiming for progression goals.
3. It allows you to monitor your progress by encouraging you to record your activities, feelings, thoughts and actions throughout the week.
4. It gives you structure so that you know what to do and when to do it. This can help you if you're struggling to eat and sleep.
5. It can help you to aim for a positive future and know/feel that this is possible.

People who suffer from depression can feel lost and empty. They become almost robotic and this can be a serious condition. Feelings of depression should not be ignored or underestimated, so you should seek advice from a medical professional. A CBT therapist may also be able to help you get to the bottom of your depression.

Anger Management

Anger is an emotion that affects our behavior. It can sometimes explode out and cause us to become extremely irrational. Sometimes a person may suffer with uncontrollable anger if they feel they've been treated unfairly and if they feel threatened, the anger can be intensified. In some cases, anger can be a good thing, because it keeps us motivated and it gives us a sense of power, but we have to be careful because we don't want it to go too far.

Anger can result in us spiraling out of control. Sometimes anger comes from stress and this can sometimes mean we direct it to the wrong place or at the wrong people. Anger can be at different levels and sometimes we let out too much or too little. Holding anger in can be just as explosive as letting it out, because it builds up inside.

CBT can help with anger management because it can help us to take a calm approach and control this effectively. Being mindful can also help to manage and control anger, so it's definitely worth checking out chapter 10 of this book too.

CBT can be helpful when dealing with anger because:
1. It can help the sufferer determine what's causing the anger.
2. If we know what's causing the anger, we can start to

put an appropriate plan of action in place to deal with that.
3. It can help to uncover a range of techniques to help cope with any anger issues or stressful situations effectively.
4. It is goal-orientated, so it provides a focus for the sufferer to concentrate on.
5. CBT is an effective therapy for thoughts, emotions and behavior, and as anger triggers all three, it is an effective method of maintaining control while working through problems.

Anger is a common issue that can be treated quickly and effectively if noticed early on. If it's left alone, it can result in numerous issues including violent outbursts, further mental health issues, and you can even find yourself in trouble legally. This can even spread into depression as you no longer recognize yourself and dislike the person you've become. It can be a long road to recovery, but learning to talk out your worries, as well as being mindful of the situation helps.

Is CBT an Effective Treatment for Children and Adolescents?

Absolutely! CBT is not just for adults; it can be great for both children and adolescents too. There are many reasons for this, but one key reason is because it's flexible and can be offered in many different formats to suit the young person. Therapy can be on a one-to-one basis, in a group, or with parents.

CBT is a useful approach for children and adolescents because it reviews many different coping mechanisms. It provides them with the tools and coping techniques they need to manage several different situations in their life, including stress and anxiety. Young people will work towards targets, so they have clear steps to take and know exactly what to do and because they are young, it is easier for them to adopt the strategies so that they use them naturally.

Young people are often receptive to CBT because the therapist does not tell them what to do but allows them to lead and work out solutions to their problems. This can be invaluable in the future when they are subjected to stressful situations and can generally help the way they think and approach things in their life.

If a young person is suffering from anxiety, depression, anger issues, or negative/emotional behavior, then CBT can be recommended by a medical professional. It has even been recommended in cases of substance misuse or post-traumatic stress disorder.

CBT for children is usually a short-term treatment program delivered by a therapist who uses the sessions to teach CBT skills and techniques to the children and sometimes their parents. In most cases, children, their parents, the therapist, and anyone else involved in the child's life could be involved in the implementation and support with CBT.

There are many different approaches that can be used with children, so it's even more important to work with the right therapist, preferably one who has worked with children in the past. Collaboration is so important, and CBT can actually work as a type of family therapy too (Effective Child Therapy, 2019). [19]

CBT is not restricted by age and has many benefits for all. The key component of CBT is goal setting and problem-solving techniques, but first, you need to identify your problems and your core beliefs, so you can start to move forward.

Chapter 4 – What's my Problem?

You already know that you need to make a change as there's some problem in your life, preventing you from moving forward or being happy. For the next part of the CBT process, we need to work out what your problems are exactly.

Working out what our problems are isn't always easy. When we've thought a certain way or believed a certain thing for a long time, it can be difficult to see that it's causing a problem because it feels natural and normal to us. Often, we know something is wrong, but we don't pinpoint the root cause and we only touch the surface. This means that the problem recurs because the problem isn't solved.

There are a range of strategies we can use to identify problems and then we can use CBT to work on solving those problems. It's time to get to work!

Strategy 1 – Identifying your irrational and negative thinking patterns and actions with Journaling.

Identifying your problems takes time so it's important to be patient at this stage. It could take a number of weeks to identify your problems. One simple way of doing this is to use Journaling. Journaling is an important CBT technique if you need to work out what the problem is. It can help you to evaluate the extremity of your problems and how deep they run.

So, what is journaling?

Journaling is a commitment. It's a record of your thoughts, actions and feelings. It's a great way to work through your emotions, actions and thoughts. At first it is a simple record, but as you start to move on in the CBT process, it will prove to be a useful tool to reflect on how you feel, and it often helps you to pinpoint the root cause of your problems. You can describe how you feel, what caused it and how you coped with the situation[20] (Ackerman, 2019) and then when you have enough information, you can analyze this and use a range of further tools to help you take action against those.

Activity 1 – Setting up and Using a Journal

To journal, you need a notebook, or online document to record events from your days. You should set your diary up in a particular way:

At the very top of your journal page for each day, I want you to note down something you are thankful for today, so ensure you leave a prompt at the top of your diary – *Today, I'm thankful for…*

You then need to set up a table of four columns:
Event – So you can note down information about the event that triggered your reaction.
Feelings – How did this make you feel?
Actions – What did you do or how did you act in response to this event?
Thoughts – What thoughts did the event trigger?

You can note down positive and negative events in the table, but you should color-code these (black for negative and green for positive, for instance).

You should also leave a blank space at the end of your page too, so you can make a personal reflection in your journal.

*You need to use your journal every day for a number of weeks. You can assess your thoughts after one week and start to work on further CBT techniques, but you should keep on with your journaling and make it part of your daily routine.

Journaling should be continuous, but you can start to work through and assess your diary after the first 7 days. Once you have enough information, you can start with the next part of your CBT process, and identify your cognitive distortions.

What are Cognitive Distortions?

Cognitive distortions are a collective name for your irrational thoughts and negative thinking patterns. As we explore them, try to relate some of the problems you have identified as part of your journaling process to the different categories. You may also find that other issues crop up, that you haven't really identified as being an issue previously until you've read the definitions and relate how you think, feel and act to these distortions.

Cognitive distortions are key when we start to make sense of our problems as they help us to make sense of our thoughts, feelings and actions. This works hand in hand with journaling and we can identify the negatives problems and then we can start to categorize them. Once we categorize them, we can plan a course of action.

Defining Cognitive Distortions

We've already established that Cognitive Distortions are different types of automatic thoughts. When we have thought in a particular way for so long, we believe it and we continue to think in that way. That's why people who suffer from anxiety and depression have a relapse, because those thoughts and feelings don't just go away. Even if we've worked through our previous issues, we can still have doubt in the back of our mind that creeps through now and then to stir things up. That's why learning to cope is so important. It breaks the cycle, so we are less likely to fall back into old habits and patterns.

Have a read through the descriptions and examples of each below. Grohl (2016) suggests that there are 15, but in this book, we have formed ten based on his studies (Ackerman, 2019)[21]. We will use the ten we've formed below throughout this book:

1. **Filtering** - The way we filter information is complex and often we filter out anything positive and concentrate on the negative.
2. **Polarized thinking** - This is when we are defeated easily because we believe there only two options in life; we either succeed or we fail. If we don't succeed, we just believe we are failure and there is no room to grow or middle ground. Sometimes we simply don't get the desired effect because we need to work on one area, but polarized thinking again focuses on the negative aspects and accepts failure far too easily. This line of thinking

acknowledges only perfection as success, but in reality, perfection is often rare.

3. **Overgeneralization** - This is a cognitive distortion identified by Beck (1967) and this basically means that we allow one single experience to define us. This is like heading to the kitchen and a recipe not going to plan. From that point on, you generalize yourself as being a bad cook. As human beings, we learn from our mistakes and should never put ourselves in a box that prevents growth and development. Cooking is a skill and if we make a mistake, we can learn to cook better next time. That's the case with most things in life. Overgeneralization blocks us from experiencing that learning curve. This can escalate to a more extreme level and affect the way we think about or treat others. It can cause us to judge and mislabel based on generalized assumptions.

4. **Jumping to Conclusions** - This is another way that we block, and it is similar to overgeneralization, except we make judgement calls and assumptions based on nothing. This is like assuming people do not like you or judging you do not like someone without really getting to know them, or that we don't like something without trying it first.

5. **Magnification or Minimization** - This is another distortion that was identified by Beck (1967) and this is when we magnify or catastrophize an event and make it more dramatic than it actually this. This is the mother of blowing something out of proportion. When you magnify an event to this level it is difficult to see clearly because panic sets in. *Does that tiny spelling mistake in an email really mean your reputation is ruined and that your boss will sack you for instance?* Although this isn't professional, others do accept that it is human nature to make occasional mistakes. It is often how we react in response to the mistake that matters. Now, Beck (1967) looks at magnification and minimization as separate entities, but Grohl (2016) counts these two distortions together, because minimization can be just as damaging. Sometimes we minimize the positive things that happen in our life because we focus on the negative. These two distortions often work hand in hand, because we magnify the negative and minimize the positive.

6. **Personalization** -This is another distortion identified by Beck (1967) and this is when we believe we are responsible for certain things that happen. We take things personally and think that something happened because of us or someone

doesn't like us because of something we have done. Often this is us thinking irrationally.

7. **Blaming others** - We can sometimes blame others for how we feel. For example, we can say that we are in a bad mood because of the actions of someone else. In reality, only we are responsible for how we feel.

8. **Dwell on what we should have done** - Often, we have certain expectations of ourselves and we dwell on certain situations in which we don't adhere to those. We reflect on what we should have done, rather than what we did do. We can be hard on ourselves and beat ourselves up over how we should have acted.

9. **False beliefs** - Grohl (2016) talks about different fallacies that we have and how sometimes they are beyond our control, because we believe them to be true. We just accept that things are out of our control, life is unfair, or we have no luck, when something negative happens, without attempting to take back control or trying to rectify the situation. For example, if something bad happens and we think that we are fated to have bad luck and just accept that there is nothing we can do, we have already accepted defeat and we don't even try to win.[22]

10. **Assuming we are always right** - This is another attitude that can hold us back as we can miss opportunities due to being so closed-minded. We have to be willing to try new things but we also shouldn't be afraid to try again, even if something didn't work on the first attempt. Imagine you applied for a job last year, and you didn't get it. You now see the job advertised again and you really want it, but you convince yourself you won't get it because you didn't get it last time. This assumption holds us back because we've already accepted defeat. We've convinced ourselves were not going to get it, so we might apply but not really put the effort in or we might not apply at all. This is because we assume we are right – we'll never get the job.

Do any of these distortions sound familiar? With CBT, we need to take a step back, to identify and assess our cognitive distortions in a logical way. Now you know what distortions are, you can start to categorize your problems with strategy #2.

Strategy 2 – Identifying and Making Sense of Cognitive Distortions

The first step to resolving cognitive distortions is to identify what is causing us these roadblocks. This can be done with or without a therapist, although if you are having trouble identifying and categorizing your problems at first, a therapist can help you to do this.

You should now have your journal and you will have filled this with at least 7 days of content, so you have an idea of the kinds of problems you face.

You should now focus on the events that initiated a negative feeling, thought or reaction, and attach them to one of the ten cognitive distortions that we've discussed earlier n this chapter. You then need to analyze these distortions in a logical way.

What evidence suggests this? What are my distortions based on? You might surprise yourself here because you may have more negative thought patterns than you think. You really need to put on your objectivity hat at this point and you can start to unravel those thoughts and begin to set goals to change these beliefs. Once you identify the problematic areas and approach them in an objective and logical way, the easier it becomes to challenge them and change them. Don't hold back!

Activity 2 – Making Sense of it all

Take your journal, and highlight all of the negative thoughts, feelings and actions that you've identified.

Make a table (you can draw this or create a digital/printable document) that includes the following columns:

Event	Feeling/Thought/Action	Cognitive Distortion	My ideal
Ran into someone at a party who used to bully me at school.	*Felt angry, upset. Caused me to be snappy with others and leave the party early.*	*Blaming others.*	*Not to feel like I've done something wrong and should leave. I want to feel comfortable enough to stay and move on.*

You need to note down the events from your journal in your table. You have to note down what you felt, thought and how you acted as a resulted. You then need to categorize the distortion. Above we use blaming others as our cognitive distortion in the example, now this doesn't mean that the bully is blameless. Bullying is terrible, but for this exercise, if we think it's someone else's fault for the way we act/feel/think then we are blaming others. Maybe it is their fault and that's fine, but this process isn't about them, it's about you right now and how you can make a change. In the ideal part, simply make a comment on your ideal situation. *How did you want to act/feel/think?*

Once you've got them all down on paper and categorized, the fun can begin.

To start unravelling your cognitive distortions, you need to focus on the distortions that you personally suffer from and think about how these harmful automatic thoughts hold you back. Look again at the example in the activity above. That person would lose out on being at the party and lose out on having fun, all because of events from the past and one person. Once we start to recognize our cognitive distortions, we start to understand why we feel or act in a particular way. We can also dig a little deeper to gain a more in depth understanding. Using the questions in activity 3 can help you get to grips with your cognitive distortions and really begin to understand them.

Activity 3 – Why?

Look closely at your cognitive distortions and make some notes on the following questions as they will help you figure out why you feel the way you do;
- What triggered the reaction exactly (something/one you seen, heard, a song perhaps)?
- Why do you think you think you reacted in that way?
- What's the worst that could happen if you faced this?
- What would make the situation easier for you, or ease your worries?

The whole strategy of identifying and making sense of your thoughts, actions and feelings is generally an effective method of therapy because you can do this in your own time and at your own pace. Once you change your frame of mind, become aware and use logic to assess your distortions, you are left with the ability to do this regularly and it will become a natural process. This is an easy maintenance strategy as you can continue to do this for as long as your journal, but hopefully your negative events will become less and less.

Cognitive distortions are a habit because our mind gets used to reacting in these negative patterns. Because they are automatic it can be tricky to see how we *should* react, because we react first and think later. CBT techniques are great at helping you to recognize those patterns and feeling able to challenge or change them. As human beings we learn things all the time, so programming our mind to think or react differently is possible. We just have to learn the skills.

Chapter 5 – Going Deeper into your Problems

You've identified your problems and that's a big step, so you should give yourself a pat on the back. Chapter 4 was a heavy chapter that focused on finding your present problems which is great. CBT focuses on the now, but you have to remember that every problem has a cause and sometimes that cause is deeper than you think.

In this chapter, we're going to focus on identifying and assessing problems that link to the way our body reacts, and we'll also consider how problems link to the beliefs we have. It's important to know the nitty-gritty before you devise a plan of action to overcome these. It's about raising awareness for now, so that you can bridge the gap between your problems and how they can have a deeper meaning.

Strategy 3 – Identifying, Assessing and Challenging Bodily Reactions

We have bodily reactions when we are sick, stressed or depressed. We've also talked about the bodily reactions we face when we suffer from a panic attack. Think about how your state of mind is affected by your negative behaviors or thoughts... Well it can also affect our body and cause a reaction. Sometimes when we assess our problems, we don't consider the impact it has on us wholly.

Sometimes events that trigger feelings, thoughts and reactions can affect our appetite and sleeping patterns, we can feel or actually be physically sick from the pit of our stomach, or we can even bring on our very own stress headache. *But why?*

Well, the body is a funny thing and like our mind, we sometimes have very little control over how it responds to certain situations. It's time to assess how our body is affected by the way we feel so that we can change. CBT is not only about changing the thoughts and the way we feel, it's about changing behavior too and the impact that all these things have on us. It's an all-rounded approach, that focuses on tackling all issues and encourages you to make choices that are better for your state of mind and health.

Activity 4 – How to Identify your Bodily Reactions

1. Reflect back on your journal, and your work from activity 2.
2. Pick 2 or 3 key events that had the most distressing impact on you.
3. Note them down in a notebook, in the back of your journal or a separate piece of paper and approach each event in turn.
4. Think about this event and focus on how it made you feel, what it made you think and how you reacted. Now, think about how your body reacted and write this down. Did you keep thinking or reliving this event in your head? How long did the reaction last for (minutes, several days...)? Note down your responses.
5. Repeat step 4 for each key event you've noted down.

Sometimes our reactions last for 5-minutes, while others play on our minds and affect us for a number of days or weeks, so it's important to pinpoint this. Maybe it's still bothering you right now.

This strategy can be used alongside both your journaling and when you're resolving your cognitive distortions. Again, it's about recognizing how your body is affected in the first instance, and then afterwards, it's about assessing and challenging those reactions, so you can think about how you can remedy them.

Don't underestimate the power of identifying, assessing and challenging your bodily reactions because it can be a powerful journey that can hit you in an emotional way. If you're ready, it's time to take your first step.

You've identified your bodily reactions to different situations and that's certainly the first step. Awareness is important because if you want so to stop feeling, thinking and reacting differently, you need to recognize what is wrong to enable you to make a change.

Now, it's time to assess and challenge those reaction, based on what you now know. The good thing about this strategy, is that it's personal to you. Sometimes people who feel stress, anxiety and depression can make themselves ill without realizing it, so assessing and challenging your reactions isn't always easy.

Activity 5- Assessing and Challenging your Bodily Reactions

Throughout the course of this activity, you will need to reflect on what you know from activity 4.

*Analyze
Look for patterns and correlations between the way you think, feel and act, to the way your body has reacted. For example, if you were put in a stressful situation more than once, take yourself back to that day of the event and the days that follow and ask yourself the awkward questions:
How did my body react?
How does that correlate with the next event?
How was my appetite?
How did I sleep?
How was my mood/stress-levels?
Was I depressed/anxious?
Did I feel unwell/tired/unsocial on that day and the days that follow?
Is this normal for me?
How was I the day before this event?
When was I next/last happy?

Make some statements about your reactions to summarize your bodily reactions.

For example, every time I become anxious, I don't sleep and become unsocial, so I shut myself off from the world to regroup my thoughts. OR, every time I'm stressed out, I become moody and lose my appetite for 3 days.

> ***Challenge***
> You have started to recognize that your body reacts in a particular way to certain events. You can use this to your advantage by challenging and targeting your reactions.
>
> If we use one of the examples from above:
> *Every time I become anxious, I don't sleep, and I become unsocial, so I shut myself off from the world to regroup my thoughts.* There are four problems – the anxiousness, the lack of sleep, being unsocial, cutting ourselves off from the world. Why (and other problem questions) is always a good place to start. *Ask yourself why we feel or react in this way? What is it that we fear?*

By asking probing questions, we're challenging our reactions and although this may not remedy the immediate issues, being aware helps because we begin to understand why we react, feel and think in a particular way.

The purpose of activity 5 was not change those bodily reactions (at least not just yet) but to analyze and challenge them. Awareness is everything and it allows us to understand our own thoughts, emotions and behaviors, which is the first step in remedying issues.

In relation to activity 5, if we did not become anxious in the first place, we would not trigger the bodily reactions such as sleep issues, and the need to be unsocial. That means we can target the problem at its core.

Chapter 3 has already talked through anxiety and anxiety disorders, phobias, PTSD, OCD, Depression and Anger. Each of those conditions can trigger bodily reactions but they can also be targeted using CBT strategies. If you feel stressed, your mood dips, or you don't sleep well, strategies such as relaxed breathing, muscle relaxation are discussed in chapter 7 and they will be great for you. Other techniques such as assertiveness and awareness training are covered in chapter 9, and you should also check out Mindfulness Based Cognitive Therapy in chapter 10. All of the strategies covered in this book, will help you to address the bodily reactions that you've recognized here.

Strategy 4 - Assessing Problem Causes Using the ABC Model

The ABC model is instrumental in CBT because it was one of the very first strategies to be introduced. You may have heard this mentioned earlier, in chapter 1 as this model was created by Ellis (1957 but it's certainly an effective model to use if you want to identify begin to understand and change your own behavior. In this section, we are looking at the ABC model to raise awareness of the beliefs we might have that influence our negative thoughts. In chapter 6, we will push this further and challenge our whole belief system.

The ABC Model is based on behavioral therapy, and again,

you can use a worksheet or table to record your problematic areas and to recognize the impact they have. We are programmed to react in a negative or irrational way, and the idea behind the ABC model, is to challenge our beliefs and the way we think.

To use the *ABC* model effectively, you need to use the first column to highlight your Activating event or objective situation. This means that you note down an event that happens that leads to a highly emotional response or causes you to think negatively. In the second column you need to write down the details of your response down - say what happened and how you feel. This will represent your beliefs and what you believe about yourself or your problem. In the final column you should discuss the impact. Here, you should bridge the differences between the initial event and the distress it causes you:

Look at the table below to see an example of how a single event can cause an irrational belief and this can mean result in negative consequences. It is important for us to make a change and turn that negative or irrational belief, into something rational. Then we can start to behave in a positive way. If we behave in a positive way to a bad situation, the more likely we are to succeed in the future.

	Irrational	*Rational*
A - Activating Event	Failed driving test	Failed driving test
B - Belief	Must pass the driving test on the first attempt.	<u>Would like</u> to have passed the driving test on the first attempt.
C - Consequence	Negative feelings of sadness, depression, anger, worthlessness.	Healthy feelings of sadness, and disappointment. Feeling of determination to pass next time.

It is important to remember that we have healthy core beliefs as well as the irrational ones and sometimes irrational thoughts comes naturally to us. They fuel our recurring automatic and intrusive thought patterns and this an impact on our state of mind. It is common to assume that we have to pass our driving test, or any test for that matter, on our first attempt. Although this would be encouraged, there is nothing to say that we should give up or cannot try again as sometimes we accept defeat and assume failure. This is a false belief. As human beings, we tend to fill our heads with false beliefs that only end up holding us back in the longer term.

If we are consumed by feelings of sadness, depression, anger and worthlessness, we will never feel good enough to pass the test and this will lead to anxiety, depression and stress because those negative feelings consume us. If we accept that we did not pass, we can start to move forward. Sure, we will be sad and disappointed initially, but we can use those feelings to fuel determination. Determination motivates us and encourages us to work harder and smarter.

In the activity below, we will use the ABC model to assess our thought patterns and raise awareness of how our personal beliefs can trigger irrational thoughts and hold us back.

> **Activity 6**
>
> For your next activity, you should make your own version of the table above and use some of the events from your journal and assess them, based on the ABC Model. 2-3 events will be sufficient to begin with, because for now, we're simply raising awareness of our beliefs rather than changing them.
>
> Detail the activating event and then your beliefs on a rational and irrational level. Be honest with yourself when it comes to your irrational feeling. You will already be aware that this is irrational, but you can only challenge this in the future if this you are honest.
>
> You then need to detail the consequences. *What are the consequences of your irrational thought? What are the consequences of your rational thoughts?*
>
> *Repeat this sequence for some of the other events in your journal and then examine your responses in the table. *Can you see how our beliefs hold us back and stop us from moving forward?*

Now that you have started to dig deeper into your thoughts, you will begin to understand how our thoughts, feelings and actions are triggered and how there can be a much deeper root cause that stems from our core beliefs. This helps you to define your problems.

Defining Problems

Defining your problems is a key process when you dig deeper and by following the ABC Model, you have already started to do this. CBT is a lifestyle change and although it focuses on the now, it's still important to look at the root causes of your problems.

You should continue with the ABC Model and working on your journal throughout your CBT journey. Don't forget to review your main issues and assess your problems as this will allow you to target them by setting goals, which we will focus on in chapter 7.

The ABC model outlines two types of negative thinking patterns; rational thought which are healthy and irrational thoughts that are unhealthy. We are not robots, so it is healthy for us to feel emotional, to react irrationally and to think negatively from time-to-time but you need to ensure you are aware of these patterns and reacting in a reasonable way. Defining our problems and challenging their root cause prevents us from amplifying issues. It's important that you can differentiate between the two, in order to define your goals effectively.

Once you have defined your problems using your journal and the ABC model, you are ready to really start challenging your core beliefs.

Remember, you are making a transformation here, so be patient. It's really important that you use probing questions to assess your own behavior, thoughts and feelings. To investigate your problems further, you can ask yourself the following questions.

- How did I feel or act (think about your symptoms and the intensity level)?
- What happened to make me feel or react like that (trigger)?
- When did I feel like this and has this happened before (look for patterns)?
- Why did I feel or react like that?

You can note down your answers and keep them with your journal and the other activities you've completed while reading this book.

We will work on changing our core beliefs in chapter 6, so keep this table and apply relevant events to this model and assess them. For now, just be conscious of how your beliefs can have an emotional impact by triggering an irrational thought.

Chapter 6 - Identify and Challenge your Core Beliefs

How hard is it to change your whole belief system? Well, when you've believed something your whole life or at least for a long time, it's certainly not easy to make that change. This is why we would suggest that CBT is a lifestyle change as it's so much more than simply resolving problems. Although CBT concentrates on the now, it's still important to go back and challenge your core beliefs. You've already started to do that in chapter 5 of this book, with the ABC Model and now it's time to challenge your whole belief system. *Are you ready?*

Mistakes

Sometimes we make mistakes in our lives and we can be really hard on ourselves. It can take us a long time to forgive ourselves and this can have a major impact on us. It's human nature to make mistakes but we have to have a certain level of acceptance too. We have to accept ourselves.

How long do you punish yourself if you make a mistake?

You see, it's not the actual act of making a mistake that holds us back, it's the way we cope with it. If we don't cope well and can't accept that mistakes are human nature, it can put us off taking risks in future as we won't feel this way again. The way we think, react and feel as a result of a mistake can create a fear of failure. This fear then holds us back as we stop seeing the worth in taking risks because we are so afraid of making mistakes and this can keep us from success in the future.

The sooner we accept that we make mistakes, and change our mindset surrounding them the sooner we can move on. Mistakes can actually be a good thing from the perspective that if we are making mistakes, we are learning something.
If we treat mistakes as a learning curve, it can have a positive impact on our life. It is rare that we make the same mistake twice and next time we take a risk, we might reflect on a previous mistake which means the next time we take a risk, the more chance we have of being successful.

Success isn't meant to be easy. If it was so easy, then we wouldn't view it in such high standing. Giving up is the easy way out and by holding back because we fear the consequences of our mistakes makes us stagnant. If you accept your mistakes, learn from them, then you are leaving room for personal growth. If you do things right next time, imagine how accomplished you will feel.
What have you learned from your mistakes?

This leads us to our next strategy.

Strategy 5 - Self-Acceptance

You need to accept yourself and accept that we all make mistakes. It is natural to want to do better than we already do, but we can't be the best in all areas. We have to have a certain form of acceptance. We can make improvements and we can play on our own strengths. Sometimes we wish we could do something else or be someone else, but it has to be within our remit and capabilities. Disappointment is normal!

> **Activity 7 – Self-acceptance exercise – Taking your own Advice**
>
> Look at your journal and reflect on one mistake you've made, or something about yourself that you don't like. This should be a something that really stands out for you and has instilled some fear. *You never want to experience that feeling, thought or action again!*
>
> Imagine that a friend or family member feels like this or has made this mistake and they're distraught. What advice would you give them?

The purpose of activity 7 is to recognize what advice you would give another person, so you can see how harsh you are being on yourself. We often think or feel things about ourselves, or act in a specific way but we beat ourselves up and blow it out of proportion. In hindsight, you won't be the first person who had that thought or made that type of mistake and you certainly won't be the last.

How would you feel if you found out that at least 5 other people you know have felt or acted that way or made a similar mistake? Imagine that this includes the most confident person you know and wouldn't expect. *What if you found out, they felt or acted in exactly the same as you did, but they handled it differently?*

In truth, many people (if not all) will have experienced the same things. The only thing they did differently, is own their mistakes or feelings.

Owning up to how we feel or what we did is a tool we can use to do better next time by thinking about what we might do differently. We can then show acceptance and move on. The others who experienced the same feelings as you didn't dwell on what they should or shouldn't have done and allow their feelings to turn into fear. They simply learned and moved on and you can do the same:
1. Go back to your answers from activity 7.
2. Note down what you would do differently.
3. Admit what you did 'I did [this]...' Come on, say it out loud!
4. Ask yourself, what have I learned from this?
5. Fill in the blanks and repeat this mantra, several times if need be: *I did [action/mistake/feeling], but it's okay because I've learned [what have you learned?] and next time, I'll do [what will you do differently].*

When you come to terms with your own mistakes, feelings and actions you can use it to your advantage. Many inspirational people in the world reflect on past experiences to help others. A business owner might speak at an event and tell you everything they did wrong, before they did something right.

The things we experience in life are a learning curve as they help us grow and reflect. It's time to ditch that old negative belief we have when it comes feeling like we've made a mistake or have acted inappropriately. Our experiences can sometimes be painful, but they can also indicate strength and shape us a person.

Keep repeating your own personal mantras for each experience in your journal when you have struggled to accept yourself or a mistake, until you have addressed each of them. You can work and build on these and turn them into something positive.
If we use them in the right way, we can even use them to motivate and inspire!

Core Beliefs

Your core beliefs are at the heart of everything you do. We can't help but to live by these beliefs because we strongly believe in them, either consciously or subconsciously. They stem from our past and they influence the way we view the world, the people in it, and how we live our lives.

Our core beliefs are often instilled inside us, but have you ever thought that they could actually be holding us back? Unraveling your core beliefs can take time, much more time than it can to unravel a problem and it also takes some time to reprogram them too as they usually all link together and they challenge the way you make sense of everything.

Our core beliefs are split into three categories; the beliefs we have in ourselves, the beliefs we have in others, and the beliefs we have in the world/life.

For example, if you think you are not smart enough to progress in your career, you might believe that others will never promote you because they don't respect you, and then you may believe that the world is against you and you'll never be able to make anything of your life.

Core beliefs of this sort are toxic because it is such an untrue and negative outlook on yourself and the world around you. This could prevent you from applying for a promotion in the future, as you will not want to take the risk due to the fear instilled. They are the root cause of anxiety, stress, depression and confidence issues. They instill feelings of worthlessness, because a person can truly believe that there's no room for growth. *But where's the proof?*

These core beliefs are completely unfounded and yet the longer we let them fester, the worse we feel. This is a form of self-torture and yet, there's no reason to do this to ourselves. Some of our core beliefs are less obvious and it can be tricky to start to recognize and unravel them. Beliefs are something we can live by since birth as they can be passed down to us. *So, how can we find out what they are?*

We've already spent time using the ABC Model to identify some of our core beliefs but there are some other techniques we can use if we're struggling to work them out. Sometimes we just have to rephrase and reframe our ideas.

We need to analyze our beliefs in more detail just like how we categorized our problems with cognitive distortions in the earlier chapters. Follow the step-by-step process in the following activity to start recognizing your core beliefs. You can use your journal or the information from the work that you've already completed with the ABC model so that you can sort your beliefs into the three belief categories (beliefs in ourselves, in others, and for the world/life)

Activity 8 – Exploring your Core Beliefs

- Note down the situation that caused your initial problem and focus on how you felt or acted. What was the negative aspect?
- Really think about what this says about you. What do you think it suggests?
- Keep asking yourself why. Why did I feel like that? Why did I act like that?
- What do you think others will think about this?
- Why will they think that? Do you have any proof that people think this or is an assumption?
- What does this mean about the world or life?
- Why do you think the world will think or react like this? Again, what proof do you have of this?
- Look at your beliefs. Are there any common themes? For example, say your beliefs all point to a lack of self-belief, that's your theme. You then need to question why you have this self-belief and form your own probing questions based on your beliefs. When was the last time you really believed in yourself? What happened to make you stop believing in yourself?

These beliefs ultimately shape the way you view the world and while some beliefs we have are fine, others can set us on a downward spiral. We need to target these assumptions and beliefs to enable us to let go of the past and move forward.

Facing Problems, Assumptions and Beliefs Head-on

If you want to face your problems, beliefs and assumptions, you must get to the root cause so that you can begin to target these. As you know, CBT generally involves targeting the present but if your core assumptions and beliefs stem from things that have happened in the past this can take a little experimentation as we aren't always clear.

To face your problems, assumptions and beliefs, we have to think about instrumental things that have happened in the past and think about how they've had a negative impact on what you believe about yourself, others and the world. Sometimes you can pin-point these yourself easily, but to get to the core, sometimes we need to experiment and record different events that provoke a reaction.

We can only target these, once we know what they are. *But how do we find out?* Exposure planning is a great strategy used to identify, challenge and monitor your problems and core beliefs. It targets the assumptions and beliefs directly and can be very effective.

Strategy 6 - Exposure Planning

Exposure Planning is a great technique in CBT that can be used to help us figure out and target our problems and assumptions. It can be effective, but it can also be quite emotional, and usually it's because of the sense of relief and realization you feel. Exposing yourself to certain situations can be an exhilarating experience. It helps you to train your mind to do something in a different way and with this technique, you get to test your own limits. It's a great way of figuring out what works for you.

This technique involves you thinking about your typical day and the type of things you do. You can make a list of the behaviors that you should be avoiding or want to change. This method is great for things like OCD because you expose yourself to the typical situation that you usually react to, but you then respond to the compulsion in a different way. Listing what you usually do shows awareness of what the problematic behaviors are, and the exposure really helps you to start coping with everyday situations differently.

Activity 9 – Plan your Exposure

- Have a look in your journal from the last week, or your ABC Model and choose some regular events that set off your anxiety or cause some discomfort or distress. It must be something that you're willing to confront.
- Look at your notes and really think about how you feel and how you usually respond.
- Think about how you could respond in a rational and better way (how do you want to think, feel, act, next time this happens?).
- What does it suggest about your problems and your core beliefs?
- Make a plan to expose yourself to a situation or event that will spark this feeling.

Triggering event	Exposure activity	Day/time of 1st exposure	Day/time of 2nd exposure	Outcome after 2nd exposure
What event triggered the feelings, thoughts and actions?	*What happened last time? What will you do to avoid or cope with the situation? How?*	*Date and time of exposure activity.*	*Date and time of 2nd exposure activity.*	*How do you feel after the 2nd exposure? Did it get easier? How successful was it? What did you do differently?*

Understanding your Assumptions and Beliefs

Once you've considered some events in your life that have had a negative impact, you then need to really think of the decisions or assumptions you make because of those beliefs.

We use our beliefs to set rules in our own lives, and they often impact on the way we react to something. If we refer back to the ABC model, we can start to think about the root cause of these assumptions and unpick our belief system. At the start of this chapter, we started to discuss the three categories of our core beliefs; the beliefs we have about ourselves, about others, about life and the world. *Just take some time to reflect on activity 9 and think about the beliefs you have that make you think, feel or act the way that you do when you encounter an event that triggers a negative reaction/thought.*

For example, if someone in your family had issues with alcohol throughout your childhood and made us miserable, we may associate this idea of alcohol and misery throughout our life. This is a belief we adopt but it's not necessarily true. This is not to suggest that alcohol is good in any way, but someone who has an occasional tipple would not necessarily spread consistent misery.

Our fear that it does, would make us avoid situations or

people involved in alcohol because we link it closely to misery, when in fact, we could find a great friend or colleague in someone that has an occasional drink. They could also be very happy and positive people but our experience and negative association forms how we think and feel about people or an occasion. Maybe we would also avoid establishments that serve alcohol if the fear grows further and this could hold us back as a result as we would miss out on social occasions too. Many people enter places even if they don't drink alcohol, for the social aspect.

Fear is something that can fuel our false beliefs. When something bad happens to us, we make certain assumptions and form certain beliefs. Often, we are prompted by fear, because we don't want to feel, think or act in the way we previously did.

It is time to start working with those negative core beliefs that are holding you back, as this will help you to improve and grow. They can be a weakness of ours and it's really important to address them and flip them around. You've already started to target your beliefs and assumptions by exposure planning, but we need to push further. Rather than feeling bad or reacting to your core beliefs, we should challenge them and think of other ways to deal with this in an open and positive way. This growth journey is much more valuable if you learn something or grow personally as a result. This is something we can be proud of!

Strategy 7 Directly Targeting your Negative Core Beliefs

Negative core beliefs are common but if you keep targeting them and challenging them, you will start to alter the way you feel. Once you have explored your beliefs and assumptions with the ABC Model, you can begin to do this.

Activity 10 – Targeting Negative Belief statements

Sometimes we believe in something and then we change our mind. For a long time, you may use a specific brand of cereal and because you believe in them, you continue to buy them. Maybe your whole family buys them, and you've never tried anything else. But you go to store to buy some, and they don't have any. You go to the next store, but they don't either, so you have to buy another. You've convinced yourself you won't like them. After lots of resistance, you try them and you're pleasantly surprised. The next time you go to the store and pick up your regular brand, you might think twice. Now, you wouldn't necessarily change your brand, but you now know the other brand is okay. It might take some time for you to make the change because habits make us comfortable. We may be more open to change now as a result of this experience - we just need to change our habit, assumption or belief.

In this activity, we're going to challenge our core beliefs, once we work them out. Going back to the driving test example, when we first looked at the ABC Model:
Belief: I must pass my driving test on my first attempt.

Based on this, our core belief is: *Failure is not an option.* There isn't a law that says we can't re-sit the driving test (or retake any test for that matter). This belief is false, it's irrational and it's unfounded. You need to respond to your core beliefs in a motivational way. Take a look at the example below:

Current Core Belief	Response to this belief
Failure is not an option	*I treat not winning or getting the results I want as a learning curve. Whenever I feel like I've failed or could've done better, I don't give up. I get back up, dust myself off, and feel more motivated than ever to do better next time.*

If a family or friend came to you with this belief, you wouldn't say *Sure, you're a failure, that's it for you now*. So, why do we do this to ourselves?

We are often our own biggest critic, when we should be a fan. We have the power to motivate ourselves and to make the change we crave.

Activity:
1. Make a table like the one above and make a list of your core values, assumptions and beliefs (you can use your journal, ABC model, or any of the earlier activities to help you).
2. Get to the heart of your core belief and find out what it really means.
3. Make a positive statement in response to each of these.
4. Display these somewhere you can see them (post it notes on the wall, your notice board, or in the front of diary). You can refer to them whenever you have doubts.

Remember, we formed our belief system in the first place, so we can change it!

Once you target your negative beliefs, you can start to cope with these better and you could even come up with strategies or ways to avoid your triggers. Having statements in response to negative beliefs is a great motivator because it really highlights how irrational we are being. They also give you a basis to start forming your new, positive and rational core beliefs.

Identifying your negative core beliefs can be daunting because we are not just challenging one idea here, we are challenging everything you believe in and sometimes we realize that those things we've lived by are unfounded and they are often responsible for our stress, anxiety, depression, behavior and negativity.

On the flip side, forming your new core beliefs can be refreshing. It can give you a new power or lease of life, and you can start to really change your outlook on life. You can do this right now! Take your table from activity 10 and form new core beliefs. Let's go back to the failing a driving test one more time: *Failure helps me grow.*

You can expand your points if you want, but this is the top and bottom of the belief. Failure helps us grow because we can learn from it, we can feel motivated and it can make us a stronger person.

This chapter is quite heavy, so if you're feeling overwhelmed right now, the strategies in the next chapter will help to calm your mind and help you refocus.

Chapter 7 – Relax, Regroup, and Believe

Are you ready to relax? The last few chapters have been deep, but you survived it and now it's time for some self-care. It's important to care for yourself, and relaxation can calm your mind and body. This is all part of the CBT process, so we're not straying from our pathway. Often, the importance of caring for oneself is not highlighted enough. We're still going to be working on beliefs in this chapter, but we're going to regroup.

To start, we're going to breathe! Of course, you're breathing right now, but we're going to learn some relaxed breathing. At the beginning of the book you were asked to approach CBT with an open mind, so even if you think this kind of thing isn't for you, you should still give it a try.

Strategy 8 – Relaxed breathing techniques

Working on your problems and beliefs can be overwhelming. It can trigger all sorts of anxiety and emotion. Relaxed breathing techniques can be used in CBT and they are particularly useful if we feel like we're on an emotional rollercoaster. They can help us to calm the mind and they can also help us to focus and think in a rational way. If we are working on our core beliefs, it's more important than ever for us to be rational. Relaxed breathing can be especially useful if you have panic attacks or anxiety disorders.

This technique may be similar to mindfulness, but you will simply focus on your breathing. As the whole of chapter 10 is dedicated to mindfulness, we're not going to go too deeply into this right now, we are simply concentrating on using breathing techniques.

Breathing techniques can help us to calm down our mind and body, and this allows us to collect ourselves and then we can reassess our problems. They are great for the present, and they can be built into our routine so that we are more likely to have a stress or anxiety-free day.

If you still aren't sure about your core beliefs or problems, you may be suffering a block. Take some time to relax and reflect, as this could help you focus and figure them out.

Activity 11 – Relax and Reflect

- ✓ Find a relaxed position in either a sitting or laying position. Make sure you don't cross your arms and legs.
- ✓ Ensure you're somewhere quiet. It can be best if you are alone.
- ✓ Close your eyes and listen carefully.
- ✓ Breathe in for 5 seconds through the nose if possible. Hold for 1 second. Then breath out through the mouth for 5 seconds.
- ✓ Repeat the process around 10 times to regulate your breathing – you should be able to hear yourself breathe. Really concentrate.
- ✓ Your arms, legs and head should all feel relaxed and heavy.
- ✓ Fall into a natural breathing rhythm and focus on the breathing and how your chest rises and falls. Do this for a few minutes until you feel calm.
- ✓ When you're ready, open your eyes.
- ✓ Stay in the relaxed position but reflect back on the thing you were doing before the overwhelming feeling kicked in. Give yourself some time to process this idea or thought again.
- ✓ If you start to feel overwhelmed again, return to the breathing technique – in for 5 seconds, hold for 1 second, out for 5 seconds.

There are alternative ways to help you control your breathing too. If you are a visual person, you can imagine images in your mind to focus on, or if you would prefer not to close your eyes, you can focus on an image. You can also play relaxing music in the background and then kick back to practice your breathing. The whole idea of relaxed breathing is to help you relax, so it's important that you find your own rhythm and do what works for you.

We all relax in different ways and when we are relaxed, we can calm ourselves and this means we tend to act in a more rational and effective way. This can certainly help if you suffer with anxiety, panic disorder and OCD because breathing can help you to cope. Being able to calm yourself helps you to maintain control. Breathing can even help with depression too (Ackerman, 2019).[23]

Now, the breathing activity is all well and good, but it doesn't explore the root of your problem or belief. The relaxed breathing technique can help you focus and encourage you to stay calm, but it's important you note this event in your journal and detail its triggers.

If you struggled when you were exploring your core beliefs, relaxed breathing should have helped you clear your mind and focus, so you can now return to that. If you managed to explore your core beliefs and you've already addressed them and written your new, positive beliefs, then you can move on comfortably to the next session, as we're going to move those beliefs from your intellect to your essence.

Move Beliefs from your Intellect to your Essence

If you want to move your beliefs from your intellect to your essence, you need to start reflecting on your new beliefs and consider the event that triggered the emotions, actions and feelings you experienced as a result of these beliefs.

Forming new core beliefs is instrumental if you want to change the way you think, act and feel. You have started to do this already, but as you continue on your CBT journey, more of these will arise, so it's important that you keep recording events in your journal, and assessing your problems, so that you can explore your core beliefs. You should continue to address the negatives by listing positive statements as you did in activity 10.

This will take time as you really need to dig deep. It is possible to make progress with self-help techniques, providing you can be open and honest with yourself and recognize your core beliefs but sometimes people choose a therapist.

You should regularly remind yourself of your new core beliefs and this is most effective if it's in a visual way. It's a great idea to note them down in your journal and remind yourself of them every morning. Alternatively, you could put them on cards and display them on your notice board, or you could create a vision board that details all of your newly formed beliefs.

Whenever you repeat your negative thinking patterns and feel like you are reverting to your old ways of thinking and acting, you need to be able to access and reflect on your new core beliefs. Really reinforce them and push the positive aspects until you believe them without question.

Once you've put your new beliefs into action and you're starting to embed them in your brain, it's time to working on flipping your negativity into creativity.

Negativity versus Creativity

Creativity is the driving force of motivation and positivity. If you typically react, or think in a negative way, creativity could be your savior. Creativity can be a therapeutic outlet within itself and there are many benefits to this. In life, we no longer have room for these negative thought patterns or reactions as our way of thinking changes. This is because we are starting to adopt our new beliefs, so we will now use our negativity for the greater good; to enhance creativity.

Being creative means to be bold, confident, and unafraid to make mistakes or fail. Creative people are driven, and never give up. Maybe you're saying *that's not me!* And right now, it might not be, BUT why can't it be you in the future?

Before you focus on transforming those negative feelings and reactions by using your creativity, we need to clear the mind and alleviate life's stresses. We are going to push relaxed breathing further, by dipping into muscle relaxation. This is a great technique that will certainly help you to clear your mind, focus on creativity and prepare you for the mindfulness work in chapter 10.

Strategy 9 - Muscle relaxation

If you enjoy things like mindfulness already, this is very similar to a mindfulness technique. We will discuss mindfulness in more detail in chapter 10 of this book but for now, we are going to focus on muscle relaxation.

If panic sets in or we are depressed, anxious or stressed, it becomes really difficult for us to think straight. When we are relaxed and can clear our mind from the daily stresses, we can start to think in a more rational and effective way. Whilst breathing relaxation can be great, muscle relaxation takes it just one step further.

Like muscle relaxation techniques, it can calm us because it too involves controlled breathing and then you begin to focus on relaxing your muscles in turn, rather than breathing. You do this until you and your body are in a fully relaxed state. Follow these steps to try muscle relaxation.

Activity 12 – Timed Muscle Relaxation

- ✓ Take yourself off to a quiet place, preferably somewhere you can lie down.
- ✓ Set your alarm for either 10 or 15 minutes.
- ✓ Tell yourself what time the alarm will sound – say it out loud and imagine the sound of your alarm in your head.
- ✓ Lay in a relaxed state. Don't cross any part of your body.
- ✓ Start breathing through your nose, in for 5 seconds, hold for 1 second, and out for 7 seconds.
- ✓ This will send a relaxing feeling through your body, allow it to flow from your shoulders, down, until it reaches your fingertips and then down your body to your toes.
- ✓ Your arms will feel heavy and you should continue to breathe, until you are in a fully relaxed state and then you can start to find your own breathing rhythm.
- ✓ Lay, in your relaxed state until your alarm sounds.
- ✓ You may wish to stay down for few minutes and refocus on your problems or issues, or you may just want to collect your thoughts.
- ✓ Take a couple of deep breaths before you sit up and ensure you move slowly, at your own pace.

This technique can help you to destress, calm your nerves and soothe your mind. A few minutes of this can help you focus on key issues and resolve them in a rational way. If you have not done this before, you can find guidance through online videos on platforms such as Youtube.

Some people prefer to be guided, while others, once they understand what they need to do, prefer to control this themselves, without guidance. You can simply use soothing music if that helps but ultimately, it is important to find the method that suits you the most, individually.

You should take time to enjoy the relaxation techniques. At the end, you still need to be able to rationalize your thoughts so you can use some of the activities at the end of this chapter to help you find solutions or change negative thinking patterns.

You will now be ready to face the world and tap into your creativity.

Turn your Negativity into Creativity

As you start to change your core beliefs, thinking patterns and actions, there's absolutely no reason why you can't be creative. Believe it or not, your experiences in life make you unique and we can use this uniqueness to spark our inner flame. You will find that the more positive you are, the better you will feel as a person and you can start to be proud as you start to work on the future.

You should always try to turn your negatives into positives, but how about turning your negatives into something creative? If you've got this far, you're ready for anything.

Here are eight ways of turning your negative feelings or reactions into something creative and positive:

- When you feel stressed, anxious or depressed, write down your causes and triggers. Use them to write a blog post or article to explain your feelings and how you coped.
- Many people use art as a way to cope and you can create something special even if drawing isn't your thing. If you feel negative, you can take yourself off to a quiet space. You can draw pictures if you like art, or you can simply color mandalas.
- Write a story, song or poem that embodies how you feel or what you know. People will find characters realistic if they are relatable, and poetry is often at its best if it's filled with emotion.
- If you're feeling negative, take some time to meditate or relax. Take a deep breath, close your eyes and think about the negative feelings or actions in your mind and then counter them with a positive statement. Write them down and create mantras and affirmations. You could even stick them around your home or office or create a book full of them.

- Dancing is a great way to express yourself. Put on a song that makes you happy and dance.
- Celebrate your goals or success stories. We don't celebrate our own achievements enough so do something to celebrate that you wouldn't usually do.
- Help someone else in a similar position. Maybe listen to someone who needs to talk through their problems or speak at a support group to inspire others.
- Be honest about how you feel to get it off your chest and then go for a brisk walk. While you are walking, you should think of five things you are thankful for.

You may even think of your own ideas here, as something positive can always come out of something negative. If we can do something that clears our mind or boosts our confidence, we may even become a little bit bolder and braver. This could instill creativity and ensure success in the future. Be as creative as possible with your ideas and find new ways to embed your core beliefs.

As well as being a talking therapy that works on solving your problems and examining core beliefs, CBT is also a goal-orientated therapy, so goal setting is imperative. Now that you know what the problems are, and you're starting to build a positive and healthy belief system, you are ready to look further into the future.

This will help to enhance your motivation as you will have something to aim for that will improve the way you think, feel and react. *That's why you're still reading, right?* Take a few moments right now to think about your ideal goal. *What do you really want?*

Be bold, brave, creative and confident. Remember, this is the new you!

Chapter 8 – Goal Setting for Greater Good

Are you ready to plan your future? In the previous chapters, we've done a lot of soul-searching by analyzing our problematic areas but now it's time to flip those on their head and start looking to the future. We're going to explore how we can set effective goals together and we'll also look at our ideal goal. But first, it's important for you to know just how goal setting applies in CBT and why it's such a key focus.

Problem Focused and Goal Orientated

The whole aim of CBT is to focus on your problems and it's goal orientated. Although it's classed as a talking therapy, goal setting is instrumental to the recovery and success of the client. It focuses on specific problems and gets you to address them directly by setting goals on how you can overcome them. Your problem can be anything that's making you unhappy in your life, from something that makes you depressed or anxious, to even getting that job of your dreams.

Whatever that problem is, CBT helps you set goals to get what you want and map out how you can get there. In the process, you identify the negative thoughts, destructive behaviors or actions and emotions that are holding you back from achieving your end goal.

There are many benefits of goal setting. To start, it gives you a clearer focus and it also helps you to understand the direction that you're heading in. This means that if you have to make decisions, you have clarity and a better understanding of what you must do. Sometimes, simply having a plan of action so we know how to get out of a certain situation or solve our problems is the key to moving forward. This can be a turning point within our therapy and is instrumental to our recovery.

It's time to spend some time thinking about yourself and focusing on what *you* want in life.

> **Activity 13 – Your Ideal Life**
>
> Before you begin reading, close your eyes and imagine your ideal life.
>
> Focus on it. Visualize it!
> *How do you feel? What changes would you need to make to get there? What problems do you want to overcome? What's your ideal?*
> You can use these probing questions to help you set your goals.
>
> *Write down three things you want to focus on achieving – Keep this for later.

When you begin writing and setting your goals, you will need to break them down into smaller stages or steps to help you stay focused and you will be able to monitor your progress as you start to reach for your overall goal. Taking small steps is often more effective because it makes the change transition smoother, and almost seamless. Keep visualizing your end goals and believe you *can* get there!

Strategy 10 – Positive Prediction Planning

Positive Prediction Planning is a great strategy that will help you get into the right mindset for goal setting. Now that you've focused on your problems, your beliefs and your ideal, you're ready to make some predictions for the future. There's only one rule – they must be positive!

Positive Prediction Planning is based on your problems. You look at your current problems, you identify what you want (your ideal or your goal, based on this particular problem) and then you predict the steps you will need to take to reach your ideal.

Activity 14 – Work towards your ideal life, with Positive Prediction Planning

Predict your future with positive prediction planning. Look at the problems you've noted in your journal and complete the table below to create your five steps to success.

What's the problem?	What do you want?	Prediction Steps to Success
I'm stuck in a job I hate and it's making me feel stressed and depressed.	I want a job that I love and will enjoy.	1. Explore career opportunities 2. Upskill or train in appropriate areas. 3. Look for opportunities and apply for new jobs, that excite me. 4. Prepare for any interviews well and boss it. 5. Get a new job that I want!
		1. 2. 3. 4. 5

You should address at least three problems here from your journal, and you should reflect on your new core beliefs and your ideal, too!

Positive prediction planning is effective at helping you figure out what you want in a positive way. It's instructional and you can certainly use this to help you form your CBT goals. If we have a problem, it's down to us to deal with it and do something about it. It's about taking the problems we face and reframing them into something positive.

Now that we are in a more positive frame of mind, it can be easier to find our focus, which leads us nicely onto our next strategy...

Strategy 11 - Finding your Focus

When you suffer from depression, anxiety disorders and stress, it can be difficult to concentrate on any one thing. That's because our mind circulates our thoughts and feelings, and it can feel quite manic and full on. It causes lack of concentration and if we can't concentrate, there's no way we can think in a rational way. We can only solve our problems and change our beliefs, if we can concentrate on the issues at hand and focus on our resolution. We should always allow time at the end of the day to reflect. This can be another way in which journaling can assist as you can write about your day and empty your thoughts onto a page before you switch off. Many people use this strategy. Even if you have all sorts to write about and it hasn't been a great day, you should always think about the positive things that have happened and really focus on how they made you feel. Be proud of those moments.

The relaxed breathing and muscle relaxation exercises from earlier in this book can help you to find your focus. As can chapter 10, when we cover mindfulness. You should also try this next activity:

Activity 15 – Epiphany Moments

Think about some of the things you would like to change from your day. They could be something negative, but to keep in a positive mindset, we should think of these as our epiphany moments. We'll call these epiphany moments, because when you acknowledge your negatives and think about what you can change, or how they could've been better, it's a light bulb moment, or an epiphany.

You did some work earlier on your ideal life. Remember, this is what you are aiming for. This is now your main focus. Close your eyes and imagine the things you would like to change from the day. They are listed behind each other and they are forming a barrier, but your goal is within your grasp, *how can you overcome each barrier?* Leap over each barrier and grab your goal. *Great, you did it!*

Now, think of how you can prevent those events from occurring again by challenging your feelings, thoughts and behaviors, using your epiphany moments. Reflect on each negative situation from your day, and imagine you handle it differently.

Close your eyes again and replay this out in your head but that you handle this in your ideal way. You're still reaching out for your goal and you're on target – you feel proud. Believe it!

Use positive phrases and say them out loud If 'this' ever happens again, this is how I will respond for a positive outcome.

It isn't healthy to dwell on the past and what you 'should' have done too much, but it's perfectly acceptable to reflect on the past and plan how we would deal with that same situation if it happened again in the future. By doing this, you are preparing yourself for the future AND you are learning along the way. You're learning that the way you reacted, or what you felt, and thought is not how you want to act or behave and with that in mind, you're planning to make that change.

Being able to focus on your thoughts and actions can help us with our future plans, and it can help us determine what we want in life and who we want to be. When our mind is full of everything, including thoughts of regret (because we should've acted differently), it clouds our judgement and it's impossible to think straight.

Finding and regaining our focus allows us to be rational and logical. When you can think and act in such a way, you've adopted a positive mindset, and you're ready to start setting your CBT goals.

How to set Effective Goals

We've already talked about CBT being a goal-orientated therapy, so we need to start thinking about the progress we want to make. It's not always easy to set goals that are personal to us, especially when they relate to our feelings, behaviors and thoughts. Regardless of how we feel, goal setting is vital in CBT and it's something that we must do as objectively as possible.

In order to set goals, you should reflect on your new core beliefs and problems that you have worked on in the earlier chapters. You can also reflect on your work from this chapter.

As you've already done the background work, things should run smoothly. We must approach each of your problems and beliefs in turn. Afterwards, we must reflect on them, their causes and how they make you feel or act.

Once you know your ideal and what you want, you need to think about how you can get there, and this is when you need to start setting goals on PAPER strategy. **PAPER** is the acronym you should use when writing down your goals.

Your goals need to be:
Precise - Your goals need to address the situation at hand, and they need to be precise, so that you are clear on what you need to do exactly.
Attainable - Your goals need to be attainable. While I believe everyone should aim high, it still needs to be possible.
Proportionate - Your goals need to be proportionate so that you can monitor and measure them. If your goals are in

proportion, it becomes easier to create the steps or stages you need to achieve your overall goal.

Effectively-Timed - Everyone can be eager to achieve their goals, but it is important to give your goal a timescale and it should be effective. For example, it would be no good to expect to start a new job tomorrow if you just applied today. Give yourself enough time, but don't be too evasive.

Rational - It can be difficult to be rational when you are acting or thinking in an irrational or negative way. Your goals need to be real for you and they need to embody exactly what you need to overcome your current thinking patterns.

When you set your goals, you should use the PAPER framework, to ensure you have tangible, clear goals that you can follow and measure.

Top 3 Tips for Goal Setting

Before you set your goals, you need to think carefully as there are some common mistakes and assumptions that people make when goal setting. This can make your goals counterproductive as rather than motivating you, they overwhelm you:

1. Try to use your newly found focus from the last section and create 3-5 goals. Although it's tempting to create lots and lots of goals because we want to do or change so much, this can actually set you back. You

can goal set at any time, so once you achieve one of your goals, think of another.
2. Remember that you don't have to achieve the whole goal at once. Make sure your objectives/steps towards achieving your goal are small and clear. Take it easy, and don't try to run before you can crawl!
3. Remember this isn't a race! Any progress is better than standing still or going back over. Some people stress if they don't make the progress they want in the desired time, but if you're going to stress, it will only hold you back. Take some time to relax and refocus. Then you can dust yourself off and try again.

Activity 16 – Set your PAPER goals

Based on your overall problems and beliefs so far, set 3-5 CBT goals using the PAPER framework, and 5 objectives or steps you need to take in order to reach your goal.

GOAL	STEPS/OBJECTIVES
1.	i) ii) iii) iv) v)
2.	i) ii) iii) iv) v)
3.	i) ii) iii) iv) v)
4.	i) ii) iii) iv) v)
5.	i) ii) iii) iv) v)

You should keep your goals somewhere you can access them easily, like your journal for instance. You can note down relevant dates in your diary, and plan how you will achieve your objectives in advance. For example, if you are wanting to overcome a specific anxiety problem, you may plan your exposure planning activities in your journal/diary too, as well as noting down any results, thoughts, feelings or actions.

Objectives can be really useful as they give us the smaller steps we need to succeed. If you have goals in mind that are attached to your problems or beliefs but need to form your objectives/steps to success, targeting your triggers is a great place to start.

Strategy 12 - Targeting your Triggers

CBT involves knowing your what your problems or issues are and adopting strategies to beat them. In order to overcome our problems, we need to acknowledge and target our triggers. We've already discussed triggers, so you will already be aware that when something makes us feel anxious, there is generally an initial trigger that stirs up those feelings. If you target those triggers at the core before they become out of control, you will often find you are pleasantly surprised at the results.

This strategy involves you reflecting on times when you feel bad or react irrationally to something. You need to then dig deeper and consider what caused that to happen. They are your triggers and if you target them, you can prevent a situation or problem from occurring. The idea is to prevent the negative behavior before it reoccurs. This is great if you find yourself falling into repetitive negative thought patterns.

Targeting your triggers means that you assess each individual problem and look at different solutions for each different problem. You may find that for one of your problems, you use the exposure planning strategy, and for another, you use relaxed breathing. So, imagine that one of your problems is that you start the day off worrying; the relaxed breathing exercise when you first wake up would be great to start your day. This would calm you and it could become part of your daily routine. If you suffer with OCD and want to target an aspect of that, then the next part of your day might mean exposing yourself to an event that usually triggers that behavior.

Activity 17 – Targeting your Triggers Technique

You now need to make a note of possible ways to target your triggers. If you find a pattern repeating itself, knowing how to target your trigger can prevent any episode of stress or anxiety.

Problem	Cause/Trigger	How can I target this?	Give yourself some encouragement
Note your problem or negative behavior here	What are the causes or triggers?	Think about how you can target this issue. What's the solution?	Make a positive statement to encourage yourself – you got this!

Targeting your triggers is a powerful preventative method of dealing with your problems. We keep mentioning preparing ourselves, but if you are prepared in advance to deal with those difficult events, you can deal with them in an effective, appropriate way.

Many anxiety disorders can prevent us moving forward in our life and so can stress, or depression. They may have been holding us back for a long time already, and they are certainly responsible for stopping us from achieving our dreams. In order to keep moving forward, we need to be confident. It's only when we've started to make progress with our confidence, that we can start to build on our awareness and assertiveness skills.

It's time to step things up!

Chapter 9 – Other CBT Techniques

We love CBT because it's continuous in our life. We can keep using its strategies in everyday life and it become natural to us. CBT is so much more than therapy and even when you've started working on your problems and beliefs, there are still further CBT techniques you can learn. We are going to review two further techniques in CBT that will empower you and reinforce your confidence.

Assertiveness in CBT

In CBT, it's important to be assertive. Many people confuse assertiveness with being forceful and it's not the same. Being assertive means that you are brutally honest, and you are willing to express your thoughts, feelings and opinions to others. Maybe this doesn't sound like you right now, but this is something that you can work on. Being assertive can be crucial in CBT because it actually helps us to maintain positive relationships with our peers and family members because it opens up communications channels.

If you bottle things up, they become problematic and chip away at us. As a human being, it is our right to voice our opinion, our concerns, and express how we feel. We shouldn't be ashamed of this, as many successful people are noted for being honest, authentic, and for knowing what they want. Yet sometimes, some people shy away from these abilities. This can be due to numerous issues, such as low self-esteem and lack of confidence.

Being assertive actually gives a sense of confidence as it validates our beliefs and opinions. CBT can help us focus on maintaining healthy relationships and being assertive is key to this. A key part of having a healthy relationship is honesty, *but how can we be honest if we can't express how we feel?*

Being assertive can show confidence and self-belief, but that doesn't necessarily mean that we are no longer approachable, or open to new ideas or opinions. When we're assertive, we don't suddenly lose our listening and communication skills. An assertive person is happy to listen and even empathize with another person, but they are not afraid to say what points they agree with and what points they don't agree with.

Being assertive means that we are approachable and open to new ideas or opinions. We accept that we have different opinions to others and are comfortable in our skin, because we promote the notion that it's acceptable to think differently from others and we're not afraid to acknowledge that.

If you aren't very assertive right now but would like to be, there are some things you can do to increase this

Five Top Tips to increase your Assertiveness

1. Actively listen to others.
2. Accept that others may have different opinions and points of view to you.
3. Express your own points of view in a calm, clear and logical way.
4. Remain positive, open and honest throughout your communication.
5. Avoid conflict by problem solving and stay strong, stick to your beliefs. [24]

Just like most CBT techniques and strategies, assertiveness is something we should work on. You could use the exposure planning strategy, and you could respond in an assertive way to a specific situation, by expressing your opinion when you would usually say nothing or very little.

Activity 18 – Reflection

Think of two situations when you weren't assertive and note them in the table below.

Think of how you could've responded or what you could've said to assert your own point of view, in an amicable and kind way. Often, people mistake assertiveness as being forceful and sometimes even rude, but that's not the case. As assertive people, we tell others what we think in a nice way, in a way that respects their point of view but indicates our own perspectives. You have a right to have an opinion.

Event	How could I be more assertive?

Being assertive gives us a sense of empowerment. If you do respond in an assertive way, we can feel a strong sense of achievement and this can boost our confidence further. This means we become braver, and a little bit better in our attitude when it comes to striving for our goals and getting what we want.

Awareness training is another improvement method when it comes to CBT as it can help you strategize and become the person that you want to be.

Awareness Training

Being aware of CBT is important, as in order to use it, you need to have awareness of what it is and how it can help you. By now, the earlier chapters will have already helped you to increase your knowledge and understanding of CBT and the relevant techniques available to you. This means you are already building an awareness of CBT, but it's important to be aware of when you need to use CBT, and also what your triggers are. This means knowing yourself, and your own conditions.

If you are a regular sufferer of anxiety disorders and depression, you will be aware of some of your core beliefs, problems and your triggers. We will discuss 4 steps to awareness training below;

1. **Identifying and Strategizing** - In the previous chapters we've focused on identifying problems, challenging core beliefs, and we focused on goal setting. This means you have already identified issues and have a strategy in place for CBT. If you haven't done this yet, you should list the things that hold you back and imagine your ideal. You should also explore your core beliefs and have created your new core beliefs so that you have a strategy to live by.
2. **Reducing and Relaxing** - Most people start CBT because they are subjected to stressful situations but

to stop the situation exploding or spiraling, you can use relaxation to reduce stress and anxiety. If you can identify those feelings of depression, stress, panic and anxiety before they start, you could relax by using deep breathing techniques (see point 4). Take yourself off somewhere quiet and relax or have a hot, bubble bath.
3. **Testing and Training** - Test and train your brain and mind by practicing the CBT techniques and strategies we've covered in this book so far. Expose yourself to the situations that usually set you off, and journal how you react, now that you're aware of your behavior. See which one works best for you and you can even tweak them so that they suit you specifically. The best CBT therapy is tailored to both the person and the diagnosis.
4. **Relaxing Breathing Techniques** - You could find somewhere quiet, lay down, and take a deep breath in, and then out for as you can and out for as long as you can then repeat for several minutes, until you feel calm. Alternatively, you could use the seven-eleven breathing techniques. In for 7 seconds and out for 11 seconds. Breathing out more than you breathe in can calm you down quite quickly and it reduce stress and anxiety. This means you can think in a more logical way.

Once you've trained yourself to be aware of your behavior and triggers, the easier it becomes to target them and take action. The most important thing at this stage is to remain patient. Not every technique we've covered will be the right technique for you and sometimes finding the remedy or treatment that works best for you takes some time.

Activity 19 – Being Aware

Just take a few minutes to note down some of your triggers and then answer the following questions:

1. Think about how you react when you are triggered – how do you feel, act and think?

2. What can you do to prevent your reaction?

3. Do you ever know in advance when you are going to be triggered, and can you do anything to stop it?

4. Is there anything you can do to avoid reacting in that particular way now that you're aware?

5. How do you think or wish you could respond when triggered in this way?

Sometimes simply being aware can stop us from blowing things out of proportion or can encourage us to think about why we react in a particular way. Just a little awareness can put a thought in our mind, and we can start to consider how we could react differently, subconsciously. Awareness shows we are open minded, and that we've started to accept our thoughts and behaviors. This is a positive step in the right direction.

There are some things to be wary of, even if you already understand and use CBT.

- Ensure you label your healthy and unhealthy emotions clearly.
- Don't lose sight of your end goal.
- Don't be fooled by your feelings or physical reactions.
- Be open minded and willing to try different techniques until you find the one that works best for you.

Being assertive and having a strong sense of awareness is a great way for you to start to explore CBT further. As you start to change the way you think, you can really start to focus on what areas of your life you need or want to improve. Training your mind to be aware is a great step towards changing the way you think, but you may want to stretch that further and look at behaviors too.

The next chapter talks about Mindfulness-based Cognitive Behavior therapy and this can help you to change behaviors while still being mindful. With CBT, it's important to explore different options and strategies to see which ones work for you. Mindfulness is great at calming yourself and your mind, which helps you to process information in a rational way, so it's worth checking out. This is especially if you enjoyed the breathing and muscle relaxation techniques.

Being mindful just means being aware of the way our thoughts, actions and emotions can affect us, and the people around us. It's the next step following awareness training!

Chapter 10 – Mindfulness-Based Cognitive Therapy (MBCT)

Do you sometimes wish you were a little more self-aware? Our mind is a funny thing as it processes information or events quickly, forcing a reaction before we've even had time to think properly. *Wouldn't it be nice to be able to put things into perspective before we reacted?* In this chapter, we're going to explore mindfulness-based CBT.

Mindfulness Based Cognitive Therapy Versus Cognitive Behavioral Therapy

We've explored CBT in detail, and we've touched on mindfulness a little, but *what is it really?*

Mindfulness has similarities to CBT, as it's described as being "a technique in which one focuses one's full attention only on the present, experiencing thoughts, feelings, and sensations but not judging them." (www.dictionary.com, 2019)[25]

Mindfulness-based Cognitive Therapy focuses on cognitive

therapy and mindfulness, rather than the behavioral aspect that we get from CBT. It looks at attitudes and mood which is why it works well for people who find themselves in severe depressive states and suffer from unhappiness regularly. Breathing and meditation is a key component of this therapy.

Mindfulness is about self-awareness in the same way that CBT is, and although CBT is hugely tailored around mindfulness, it does involve some aspects of analyzing and working on those things too, which sometimes means we judge our thoughts and feelings. CBT also focuses on the behavior aspect too and evokes change, whereas mindfulness raises awareness and believes that becoming aware itself can implement the change without forcing it. Both concepts focus on the present and try to implement changes moving forward.

By adding mindfulness to cognitive therapy, we demonstrate an appreciation for ourselves as well as showing flexibility in our thoughts. There is growing evidence to suggest that MBCT can be a beneficial treatment when it comes to mental health issues and it's often thought of being a great self-help tool (Endelman, 2006)[26]

Important ideas in Mindfulness-based Cognitive Therapy

Mindfulness-based Cognitive Therapy focuses on emotions, thoughts and attitudes. Important ideas in relation to MBCT are:

- Building up a tolerance or coping mechanism that allows us to deal with painful situations better.
- Being open and non-judgmental.
- Reaching an enhanced state of awareness.
- Allowing us to gain insight into ourselves and being in touch with how we feel.
- Using meditation techniques to reflect, recover and cope with specific situations. This can promote emotional wellness.
- Incorporating breathing techniques to help us calm down and cope with our feelings and emotions.

Mindfulness-based Cognitive Therapy is aimed at those that suffer from heightened depression regularly and its key components teach clients to make a break from those negative thought patterns and cope better, whilst improving self-awareness.

How does MBCT Work?

The aim of MBCT is to try and prevent relapses of depression. If a person suffers from regular depressive episodes, it's important to try and change this pattern. MBCT focuses on changing your relationship with your emotions. Mindfulness activities, such as meditation can help to create balance and just like CBT, you can start to change your automatic negative thought patterns and replace them with new ones.

MBCT is about creating a routine and adopting mindfulness technique to cope with an overwhelming situation. The hope is that you can replace your negative thought patterns and prevent those feelings of sadness from turning into depression (Psychology Today, 2019)[27].

Problems that may be addressed by MBCT

Much like CBT, mindfulness-based cognitive therapy is mainly used when treating depression, and this includes moods and feelings of sadness It has been recognized to help those suffering from anxiety disorders, relationship issues, pain, stress and substance misuse too. Let's not forget how useful these coping strategies are in relation to panic too.

If you start to feel down, overwhelmed, or you feel a panic attack coming on, the techniques involved in this treatment can actually prevent it from escalating into depression, although this type of therapy is usually suggested under a therapist if you suffer from depressive episodes regularly (usually three episodes or more).

MBCT Techniques and Exercises

Below are some different techniques and exercises that you might want to explore as part of your MBCT routine. Remember, routine is everything, so planning ahead in time to breathe, meditate, or exercise is a great way to start your MBCT treatment.

Breathing Exercises – Before you can meditate, you need to master your breathing. When we breathe, we typically use our chest and we raise it up and down as we inhale and exhale. Breathing from the diaphragm and stomach area is recommended with MBCT and this involves relaxing your stomach and allowing it to rise and fall as you breathe deeply. You may need to practice your breathing, daily, so spend some quiet time focusing on your breathing technique. You can lay back in the chair, close or open your eyes, or you may prefer to lie down.

Guided Meditations – Many people learn to get themselves into a meditative state without being guided, but for beginners, there are many guided meditations you can use online, on channels like Youtube. Often, guided meditations focus on a specific area, but there are ones that focus on sadness and depression. If you're going to try guided meditation, research the different ones available and listen to them for a few seconds until you a find soothing voice. Once you've found the one for you, kickback and relax. You should practice your breathing techniques for a couple of minutes, just before you begin.

Walking Meditation – With any meditation, you need something to focus on and in this case, you focus on your walking. You don't focus on each step or look at your feet, you simply focus on the fact that you are walking. Walking is a great way to clear your mind and because it's exercise, it gives you the opportunity to refocus, and you will feel refreshed.

Yoga Stretches – Yoga is a great exercise for mindfulness, CBT, and MBCT as it is already a meditative exercise. There are different types of yoga, and some are more spiritual than others. Kundalini Yoga is meditation based and involves quite a lot of breathing exercises as well as chanting. You can attend a class, or there are tutorials online too, if you would prefer.

Activity 20 – Be Brave

There are four mindfulness techniques listed above: Breathing Exercises, Walking Meditation, Guided Meditation and Yoga Exercises.

Choose one of them, preferably a technique that you've never tried before (go on, be brave).

Try it as part of your daily routine for 1 week. Remember, now that you are more 'aware' you should be able to monitor this activity and its outcomes independently, so be objective, realistic and open minded.

Monitor your progress:

Date/Day and time	Activity (what did you do?)	Outcomes: (How did you feel? Did it have a positive/calming/motivational impact? Did you do anything that you wouldn't usually do? What could you do differently? How did it help?)

Other techniques from CBT like journaling, are helpful for MBCT. Recording your thoughts shows that you're paying attention to yourself and your needs. It's a form of self-care which we could all do with a little more of.

MBCT is focused a lot more around positivity, so you could also think of some things daily, that you are thankful for (Edelman, 2006)[28]

Benefits of Mindfulness

As mentioned already, being mindful is a way to take care of yourself and this has numerous benefits for your mind and body. This includes:

- Better general health and state of mind.
- Improved concentration levels.
- Insight into one's self and more in tune with emotions.
- Better control of thoughts and the ability to think rationally.
- Stronger problem-solving skills.
- Feeling motivated and positive.
- Decreased stress and anxiety.

Mindfulness Skills

Being mindful helps us to embed many skills that can help us in our life. It can help us to process our thoughts in a more positive way, as maintaining a fit and healthy outlook. As we feel happier and healthier, we take back control of our lives and we are less likely to feel depressed, anxious or stressed.

Mindfulness can help us to appreciate ourselves and understand the importance of caring for our mind and body. When we feel motivated and content, we are able to overcome barriers that hold us back. We can also feel rested and relaxed which helps us to think rationally.

This means that we often live for the moment and live a happy, fulfilling life!

Other Alternative Cognitive Behavioral Approaches

There are several alternative cognitive behavioral approaches that you can consider:

Acceptance & Commitment Therapy - ACT is different to CBT because rather than challenging negative thoughts, it encourages you to accept your thoughts and then you use something called diffusion techniques to help you overcome these thoughts. You use three broad categories of techniques, the first being acceptance, the second is mindfulness, and the third is based on your commitment to your values. Values give us a purpose, allowing us to reflect on what is really important to us in life (Hayes, 2005)[29].

With this type of therapy, you can still set goals to move forward and it's suggested that knowing our values can free you from the stresses in your life.

Dialectical Behavioral Therapy - The main goal of Dialectical Behavioral Therapy is to gain balance as you expose yourself to difficult emotions by recognizing and experiencing them, then you aim to make a positive change to your behavior.

This therapy is closely linked to CBT as you still set goals and it's aimed at people who feel intense emotions and react in a damaging way. The most important thing is to accept yourself and your reactions, and then try to change these negative or harmful behaviors (Mind.org.uk, 2017).

By talking with a therapist, you can gain an understanding of why you feel and act the way you do, which is part of the acceptance process. It's only when you've taken the first step of 'acceptance', that you then become ready to make those positive changes and move forward (Mind.org.uk, 2017)[30].

Meta-Cognitive Therapy - Meta-cognitive therapy was initially designed to treat generalized anxiety disorders. This refers to metacognitions, which are claimed to be the aspect of cognitions that actually control our thinking process. They refer to negative thinking patterns as being Cognitive Attentional Syndrome and they are driven by underlying positive or negative beliefs. The therapy then focuses on challenging and removing the negative beliefs. It can help you gain control of your thoughts by raising awareness and it helps you to cope with negative ideas and thinking patterns.
We can be trained to use our metacognitions to retrieve our memories, but they generally operate in the background. By the end of the meta-cognitive treatment, you can have a more flexible response.

There are many different types of therapies, techniques, and treatments when it comes to Cognitive Behavioral Therapy and we've also explored related therapies too. The most important thing is finding an effective treatment or therapy that suits your needs and symptoms. Sometimes, you may wish to try different techniques until you find the one that fits you best.

Once you find the right treatments, techniques or therapies, and you start to make progress, you need to start thinking about integrating CBT into your daily life and maintaining the momentum to ensure you don't slip back into your own ways (Caselli, 2019)[31]

Many people find that in the initial stages of CBT, they need some assistance with the practices and therapies. Sometimes, they even hit a roadblock when they've made some progress. There's no right or wrong time to change your CBT therapy or treatment. Again, this is individual to you, and your needs. In the next chapter, we get a little philosophical as we look at different treatments for CBT and talk through the details of a complete treatment program. We'll also reflect on therapists and how they can help you make progress and move forward.

Chapter 11 - CBT Treatment

In this chapter, we will explore different CBT treatments and answer common questions on CBT methods and therapy sessions. If you're not quite sure if CBT is right for you, this is the section for you. We'll also think about what you should expect.

How will I know if CBT is for me?

You probably won't know for sure if CBT is for you until you start practicing it. There are some indicators that it might be for you, if you resonate with the points below.

CBT may be for you if:
1. *You like to have something to focus on and a clear direction.* CBT is orientated around personal goals that target the problems that you personally identify. If you like to know what you are aiming for and you need key points to focus on, then CBT could be the treatment for you.
2. *You are willing to learn and work on new techniques and methods.* CBT is a huge learning curve. You learn new techniques, about your fears and beliefs

and sometimes you make realizations about yourself that you didn't previously know.

3. *You're ready to work on the present, not the past.* CBT largely focuses on the present and future. As you know from the earlier chapters, you are required to do some digging into your past when you explore your negative core beliefs.

4. *You are ready to make a lifelong change in the way you view life, yourself and others.* CBT isn't a quick, overnight fix. It requires you to carry out self-reflection and a lot of work on yourself. It becomes a new way of thinking, as your thought patterns change and evolve in a positive way.

5. *You are open minded.* It is important to be open minded when it comes to CBT. There are occasions when you might think that specific activities are not for you, are similar to a previous activity, or you might just not want to try them for one reason or another. The best think you can do is swallow your pride and just give it a try. You have nothing to lose and you never know, you might surprise yourself.

You like simple, yet highly effective ways of solving problems. CBT is simple, yet extremely effective. It focuses on resolving issues, beliefs, feelings and thoughts, by targeting negative patterns. There is a lot of research to support CBT methods, some of which we've reflected on in the earlier chapters. Cognitive and behavioral techniques have been used for decades, and it is now a recognized therapy for stress, anxiety disorders, depression and so much more. (Smith, 2018)[32]

Do I need a Therapist?

This is a tough question as only you can make this decision. With CBT the treatment is individual, and people approach it in many different ways. Many people manage CBT alone and are happy with the difference it makes in their lives as they adopt new strategies, but others may struggle. If a person has severe confidence issues, suffers with depression or an extreme form of anxiety (or other issues), they may not be able to start CBT without some help and may opt for a therapist.

There isn't a right or wrong time to choose a therapist with CBT either. Often, people start practicing CBT techniques, but they then become stuck and are unsure of how to move forward. If this is you, then you may find a therapist instrumental in your therapy.

A therapist will challenge you and ask you those awkward questions. They will also challenge you and help you to figure out the best forms for treatment for you. They also hold you accountable, so if you work best in this way, a therapist could be just what you need. The most important thing is to enlist a therapist if you want or need one as you should never be afraid to get the help or assistance you need, whether it's long or short term – your choice!

What Should I Expect on my First Visit with a CBT Therapist?

Your first session with your therapist is really to find out if your therapist is the right fit for you, and you are the right fit for them. It's a time to be really honest, and sometimes in order to feel that way, you need to have a solid connection.

Your therapist will want to know what you expect from the sessions and what aspects of your life (emotions, behaviors and think patterns) that you want to change. They will also want to know about the things in your life that you don't want to change too. It's worth having a think about these and any barriers you feel that you face in your life (that you are aware of). It's worth thinking about these things before your session and you can even make notes.

In order to provide an effective treatment plan, your therapist will want to know about you and your life so that they can see the bigger picture. This means that during your first CBT session, your therapist will ask you a lot of questions, maybe about your personal life, social life, family, work, and education. They might also ask you how you feel about certain aspects of your life too, for example, they could ask if you are happy in your job/relationship? Or if there is anything you would change.

During this initial period, your CBT therapist will be assessing you constantly so that your treatment targets the right areas. This will help you to get the most out of your therapy. The assessment period can last for more than one session. As a goal-orientated, person-focused, therapy, it can take a little time to work out the root cause of your problems and figure out an individual treatment plan or program. (Gray, 2019)[33]

The most important thing is to create a plan that works for you, so be patient!

What Happens in a CBT Session?

CBT sessions are slightly different for everyone but generally, they are a talking-based therapy session. It can take place as a group session or as a one-to-one session and the idea is that you work with your therapist to break down your problems.

During your assessment period, you will set some goals and they will indicate what you want overall and the therapist's aim is to get you on the right path. You may be asked to keep a journal or diary to record your thoughts and actions, especially in the beginning as this will help you to find any recurring patterns. Your therapist will encourage you to lead the way and identify these yourself.

Your therapist will question you, as well as analyzing your thoughts and actions to help you solve your problems. Basically, at first, they will help you evaluate which are rational or irrational patterns. They will then challenge you and help you work out how you can change any irrational, unhelpful or negative patterns.

As mentioned earlier, you will have some end goals already, but you will need to break them down further into smaller steps. This will help you to monitor your progress during the sessions. You will spend some time at the end of your session discussing how you can put your changes into practice, and you may be left with some homework that will help you embed your new processes.

Remember that your therapist is there to support you. Their job is not to force you into doing anything you're not comfortable with. They will ask you the difficult questions and challenge you, and they could even help you unravel why you don't what to do a specific thing. Their focus is to help you make progress, or at least know why you feel or act the way you do, so that you can start to live your best life.

How Long does CBT Last and How Frequent are the Sessions?

It's difficult to put a timescale on CBT sessions because if you are continually making progress, then you may want to continue with the sessions over a longer period of time. Having a therapist not only helps you figure out your problems, but also holds you accountable for your actions.

CBT sessions are tailored for the individual and they typically last anywhere between 30-60 minutes. People generally either choose to have weekly or biweekly sessions with their therapists and while some people may only need 5 therapy sessions, others could have around 20.

If you find that you are getting towards the end of your therapy, but you still feel like you need accountability or someone to chat to from time-to-time, there may be other options. Maybe you could buddy-up with someone and then you can support and motivate each other.

How do I Find the Right CBT Therapist for me?

Finding the right therapist can be daunting. You could be referred through your own doctor, or you could search yourself for a private practice in your local area. The best thing to do when searching is to call them and have a chat about what they can offer you. Some therapists offer a free first session or telephone consultation, so you should take advantage of these offers.

It is extremely important to have a good therapist-client relationship and in order to do so, you need to choose the therapist. While medical professionals may be able to recommend someone to you, it is worth remembering that there are many different types of therapy. Different therapists might specialize in different types of therapy so you should consider this when you are searching for your CBT professional.

A CBT therapist should be qualified to ensure you get the best from your therapy. CBT professionals are usually qualified Counsellors, Psychiatric Nurses, Psychiatrists, or Psychologists. You could also search for a therapist by looking through directories but ensure that they are qualified, accredited, or licensed professionals.

Medical professionals are ultimately the best place to start when searching for a therapist as they can provide you with recommendations for legitimate therapists. You will only truly know if you have found the right therapist when you work with them. At your initial consultation or when you first make contact on the telephone, you should be honest about your needs and expectations. If you need intensive and regular therapy but it turns out your therapist can only fit you in once per month, you're not going to get the therapy you need. You should also discuss costs, payment terms, and ask how long your sessions will last as well as treatment timeframes. You may not know exactly but having a rough estimate is useful.

Why do I Need to have a Good, Collaborative, Therapeutic Relationship with my Therapist?

When you choose a therapist, it is important to set some ground rules and agreements. If you have the right therapist, are clear of what you expect from your therapy, make agreements and set ground rules, to ensure that you get the best possible outcome.

You could be asking yourself, why you need to have a good, collaborative relationship and basically, this is because it will ensure you succeed.

Therapy is not a one-way street, as each person must commit and do their part. If you and your therapist don't have the same goals in mind, don't agree, or aren't committed to the therapy, then your therapy may not be a success. Ensure you are aware of the roles and responsibilities of both the client and therapist. Your therapist is there to hold you accountable, to help and support you. They should help you implement CBT techniques and give you the tools or information you need to change your behaviors. They will have knowledge and experience of many different techniques, but they should also be honest and realistic, while ensuring you stay motivated.

Your therapist is not there to do the work for you or tell you what to do. They can advise and give their opinion, but they want you to take ownership. You both need to have respect for one another and be committed to the therapy. Remember a good therapist will challenge you when and as they feel it's necessary!

Will the CBT Therapist be able to Understand and Appreciate my own Background?

When you first started reading this book, you were asked to remain open minded. Your therapist will (and should) return this – they will be open minded, and they will appreciate your background.

A good therapist will have excellent listening skills and they will come from a therapy related background; maybe they'll be a psychologist, psychiatrist, or counsellor, but they will have trained and specialize in CBT. They will have dealt with various people from a range of backgrounds, and as a professional, they will understand and appreciate you as an individual.

Your therapist will have worked with others previously, with similar problems and they are trained well to help you deal with your thoughts, feelings and actions effectively. They will be non-judgmental, and extremely knowledgeable in their field. Make sure you chat to your therapist and you should also do some background research too. Don't be afraid to check their qualifications, licenses, and other credentials.

Activity 21 – Assess the pros and cons of hiring a therapist

We've established that it depends on the individual, whether or not a therapist is required.

Reflect on your own problems and beliefs with CBT in mind and highlight the pros and cons of having a therapist.

Belief or Problem	Therapist Pros	Therapist Cons

What about medications?

Again, CBT is tailored to the individual so there's no way to answer this. Medication advice should be taken from a medical practitioner only. There are people who are not keen on taking medication, and they've decided to start with CBT. It's good to stay mindful of this and never rule it out. If a medical professional says we need medication, then the chances are, for now, we need it. There are many different points of view when it comes to medication and it is important to remember that if you have been prescribed medication by a medical professional, you should never stop taking this in favor of CBT without seeking proper medical advice from a qualified person. Reducing or increasing medication is dangerous and should only ever be done under guidance from your doctor.

Some people try CBT as an alternative to medication or as well as medication. CBT can work in both cases, and it is possible that CBT can help you reduce your medication in the future, but this should again, be under medical advice. Your doctor only prescribes medication that is suited for you, and we have to remain open minded when it comes to medication as sometimes this is necessary for recovery.

If you start using CBT but think you may still need medication, ensure you seek medical advice as it is really important to ensure you get the help you need (Branch and Wilson, 2012).[34]

Chapter 12 – Maintenance

You're done, you're better, you're cured…

If only!

Now, I know that if you are reading the maintenance stage, then you will have made great progress with CBT and that's great news.

Congratulations!

BUT now the real work begins. It is amazing that you have developed and made the progress you have so far, but you need to embed and refine CBT practices and techniques into your life and ensure you keep up with this positive way of thinking, reacting and feeling.

You have all the tools you need, so now we need to store them in our mind, so that we can utilize them whenever we need them.

How to Maintain Automatic Thoughts and Cognitive Distortions

The last thing we want is for those negative automatic thoughts to creep up on us again. CBT is not something that you should simply stop once you start to see improvements, but something you should continue to do. You should certainly keep working on your think pattern strategies.

Use journaling methods to note down your thoughts and analyze them later. *Are you experiencing any new negative thoughts? If so, analyze it – what was the trigger? Why do you think that?* You can also reflect on old ones. This is great to challenge your automatic thoughts, your beliefs and to challenge your cognitive distortions.

Put your new core beliefs into practice. You should review your new beliefs daily so you can imprint them in your mind. You should build them into everything you do. Use positive statements or affirmations that relate to your core beliefs every morning and repeat them aloud.

Breathing exercises are a great way to calm and clear your mind so that you can calm down or take a moment to process your thoughts in a rational way. We've discussed these already and they can be very effective.

Mindfulness and meditation techniques are great ways to control and maintain your automatic thoughts by helping you maintain a positive outlook that is ready to solve any problems that life throws in your direction.

Activity 22 – Reflect and Think

*Reflect on your problems and beliefs and think about how or why they may need maintaining. Think about if they are long-term or short-term issues and what you will need to do to maintain them using CBT techniques.

Find the Full and Objective Perspective

You should still continue to grow with CBT even when you've achieved your initial goals and one way you can do that is by adopting an objective perspective. This is something that you are aiming towards already, because it changes the way you think. In CBT you are taught to look at things in a logical, unbiased way,

Having a full and objective perspective means that you take an overall view of a situation and your perspective is not clouded by your emotions or how you feel. You should remove yourself from the situation, feeling or thought, and look at this objectively, whilst maintaining an unbiased and non-judgmental point of view.

Emotional Reasoning

CBT is all about reasoning with your own thoughts and figuring them out, so the next step from this is to keep challenging why you feel a particular way. Whenever you feel a strong emotion you should reason with it. *Is it rational or irrational? How is it making you feel? Why? Is that a good enough reason to feel this way?* By doing this, you stop yourself from being able to overreact, and you can take a moment to question and reason with your emotion

Forging New Synapses

You should keep practicing and questioning the way you think, even when you think you've mastered rational thinking in CBT, it's a working progress. A synapse is a way that we receive and send information in our brain. When something is an impulse, it happens quickly which means that they are difficult to control. As you start to reform your thinking patterns, you can start to reprogram your brain. Rather than negative messages, your brain (with practice) will automatically start to forge new messages and eventually, your thinking patterns and synapses will be automatically be positive.

Avoiding Backsliding

For maintenance purposes, you need to monitor yourself so that you don't revert back to your old ways. You don't want that, *do you?* Keep recording your thoughts and challenging anything negative. We all have good days and bad days, which we can accept but you must remember, a pattern is something that recurs. Staying aware of your own thoughts and feelings can just make you a little more thoughtful when it comes to your own reactions. By challenging yourself, you are keeping that sense of motivation.

Keep up CBT

You should never just stop with CBT, simply because you feel you've improved. CBT is a way of life. If you are tired, you should sleep, if you are hungry, you should eat, if it's cold outside, you wear a coat, so in the same essence, if CBT makes you happy and content, why would you stop? You can use that old excuse of not having time, but the question on your lips should be, *how worthwhile is it to stop?* If CBT has improved your life, your motivation, yourself as a person and maybe even your health and happiness, what could happen if you just stop? *Can you afford to?* Mindfulness, breathing techniques, journaling, goal setting, and meditation can actually save us time as we are less likely to feel stressed, procrastinate, and struggle with our motivation. CBT can be life changing, but you should make it part of your life and routine. It's more than just a treatment!

How your New Healthy Brain Functions

Your brain controls how you think, act and feel every day, in fact it controls everything we do and how we do it.

CBT keeps your brain functioning to the best of its ability. You will be sharp and calm, your brain will process thoughts in a clearer way and your thought patterns will be positive.
If you're also getting enough rest, your mood will improve, and you will generally feel happier and motivated.

For the final part of maintenance, you should produce your own personal maintenance plan, to help you continue on your CBT journey:

Activity 23 – Personal Maintenance Plan

*Create a personal maintenance plan for yourself.
*Ensure you set at least three goals on the areas you want to improve or develop further with CBT.
*Think about how you will build the steps towards your goals, and your maintenance techniques into your routine.

GOALS: 1. 2. 3.	
Steps for improvement/maintenance	How can I build them into my routine?

Before you finally go it alone, it's important to remember that the CBT strategies we've covered in this book, are only a taste of the benefits that CBT can have on your whole life. As a bonus, there's an extra chapter added to this book that explains how CBT techniques can be used to boost your energy.

Chapter 13–BONUS CHAPTER: Ten Ways that CBT Techniques can be Used to Boost your Energy

Everyone needs an energy boost from time to time, *am I right?*

Cognitive Behavioral Therapy certainly has many fantastic benefits, but one thing we haven't yet focused on is how you can use CBT techniques to boost your energy. We have discussed some of these energy-boosting steps inadvertently, but in this bonus chapter, we will explore how we can use CBT techniques to boost your energy and why they work.

1. Increased motivation

Goal setting can increase our motivation. This is because we are driven towards something, as we have a target that we are aiming for. Imagine we're practicing archery. Our bow is loaded with an arrow and there's a large target in front of us with a big red circle in the center. *Where do we aim?*

We're naturally motivated to aim for the target, of course. If we are motivated, then we are energized, because we're pumped – we want to hit the very center of our target. We can do this!

2. Better sleep and relaxation

Most people will agree, if you've had a good sleep or some time to relax and reflect, we naturally have more energy. Sleep improves our focus and when we are relaxing or sleeping, our subconscious is processing our thoughts, ideas, emotions, actions and events from the day. Our subconscious needs time to turn them over in our mind and make sense of everything. When we've processed everything, we're ready to make decisions or judgements, and we can also process more information without feeling overwhelmed.

3. Less Stress

If you are stressed out, your mood and energy levels are often low. Often, we can't be bothered to do very much as our emotions drain us and fatigue sets in. CBT works to help you reduce the stresses in your life. This will increase your energy levels, so make the most of them by ensuring you still use CBT techniques to maintain your well-being as this can also link to improvements in your general health too.

4. Better coping techniques

If you are using CBT techniques, you will be coping better with the situations that usually act as a blockade against you. You will have already started to embed the coping techniques that work best for you. Now it's time to push them further and use them to boost your energy levels. When you're reasoning with your thoughts, actions or emotions, remind yourself how far you've come. The prouder you feel, the better, now repeat "I'm amazing. I've come so far". *Say it like you mean it!*

5. Mindfulness and Meditation

Mindfulness and Meditation works on your mind and the way you feel about yourself. If you've been using or experimenting with this part of CBT, you will really be able to take energy boosting to the next level. Mindfulness is all about reflection and awareness of one's self, so this really gives you the time to plug your energy levels with positivity. Meditation is an amazing practice for boosting energy levels, so why not put in your ear pods, click onto Youtube and search for *guided meditations to boost energy levels* and you might be surprised with how many options are available to you.

6. Improved self-care

If we are taking care of ourselves, it shows we appreciate

ourselves, and this can boost the way we feel. Self-care is something that many people don't spend enough time on and that's because it's sometimes difficult to recognize our own self-worth. With self-care, we spend time commending ourselves or we could receive a treat as a result. Often, something simple like a hot, peaceful, bubble bath can really help our state of mind and we can feel ready to take on the day ahead. Self-appreciation certainly makes us feel good and helps us to feel worthwhile and energized.

7. Confidence Boost

A confidence boost is a great way to increase our energy levels. Confidence is a state of mind, and it's how happy we are, with the belief we have in our self. Sometimes we don't believe in our knowledge, skills or abilities and these doubts drain our mind. In comparison, when we feel confident, we have the ability to think in a logical and rational way and we are often more capable of making better decisions.

8. Impact and Exercise

It's common knowledge that exercise makes us feel more energized and this has a major impact on our energy levels. CBT suggests low-impact exercise like walking or yoga stretches, and such things can really help you boost how you feel and increase those energy levels. As you get stronger, you might exercise longer or harder and this will boost your energy levels further. Exercise is so important, and it gives us the *feel-good* factor, but we should concentrate on building our strength slowly for both our body and mind.

9. Less self-doubt is a great feeling

If you have less self-doubt because you've solved your problems and changed your thinking patterns, then you will feel a higher sense of belief in yourself. Self-belief and confidence are closely linked, but the more belief you have in yourself, the more likely you are to trust your instincts and decisions. At the beginning of this book, we reflected a lot on how we can be held back by our thoughts, emotions and actions but once you've mastered the art of dealing with those, you can push even further. That's right, it's time to take risks! I'm not talking about risks that can seriously injure you, just maybe something that you've always wanted to do, or something you've never done before because that little voice in your head wouldn't let you. It blocked you. You now believe in yourself; you trust your own judgement and you're ready to try something new. *Exciting, isn't it?* That's your energy levels getting ready because excitement makes us feel happy, ready for anything, and alive.

10. Better General Health

You can't even begin to deny that overall, CBT brings better general health. We feel good in our mind, body and soul, and we want to be healthy. When we start exercising and feeling good, we start to take better care of ourselves. I'm not just talking self-care here, I mean everything. CBT can promote a healthier attitude and a healthier you. It can encourage you to start eating healthier and again, this is down to self-worth as we start to take more pride in ourselves. CBT encourages us to take care of our mind, live our best life, and aim for happiness. It also promotes exercise and meditation and if you incorporate them into your lifestyle, you can easily find that you no longer comfort eat, crave sugar and salt, and indulge in the same fatty or sickly foods we wanted when we felt depressed. Sometimes, if you're depressed you don't eat, but CBT can encourage us to maintain a healthy balance by eating the right foods regularly in order to maintain energy levels. A healthy diet certainly boosts our energy levels and if we have good health, the energy boosts will last longer.

There is no doubt that Cognitive Behavioral Therapy can boost our energy levels, but it's down to the way you use and incorporate the techniques. Ensure that you use the techniques that are most effective for you, and ensure you keep practicing CBT for maintenance after you've achieved your goals. Use the techniques you've been learning to recognize and utilize your newly found energy. You may not have even realized that you had those energy boosts at your fingertips, but don't waste the opportunity and let them go unused.

CBT will work around you as it's a long-term way of life. Keep following and practicing because for you, it means a constant and consistent, better future.

Conclusion

Throughout this book, we've looked at some great CBT strategies. CBT is a very flexible and helpful therapy, that caters to many people. The strategies in this book are known to help with stress, anxiety disorders, and depression. If you have used the approaches in this book, there is no question that they can help you live a happier life.

This book has strategies that can certainly help you, if you are susceptible and open to CBT. The whole aim of CBT is to challenge you, explore problematic areas and beliefs, and to encourage change to any patterns that are leading to your unhappiness or distress.

CBT enables you... It enables you to grow as a person and understand the reasons why we might act, think or feel in a particular way. If the strategies and techniques are used in the most effective way, they can be life changing. However, Cognitive Behavioral Therapy isn't for everyone. It will only work if you WANT the change and are willing (and motivated) to go on this self-discovering journey.

CBT is not a magic formula and obviously, there are

occasions when it doesn't work for a person or isn't enough. You should never ignore your feelings, thoughts and actions, especially if you are a known sufferer of depression, stress or anxiety disorders (and other illnesses discussed in this book), so with this in mind, you should always seek advice from a medical practitioner above anything else.

Cognitive Behavioral Therapy makes you address your problems and maintain a healthy state of mind, so it's certainly worth trying as it can make a big difference to your life by changing your automatic thoughts. People who use CBT have become successful in many aspects of their life, because they've changed their whole thought process and have generally taken a more positive view of life and altered their mindset. This may mean we can become more successful in our career, we become happier with life, and become a better, healthier person. If you think rationally and logically, you can increase your confidence and other people will see this in you.

CBT can certainly help you fulfill your dreams and get that spark back for life. Even if you don't suffer from a diagnosable condition or disorder, you've got nothing to lose by giving it a try and it could help you revaluate your current situations and learn to live a free and happy existence.

The Cognitive Behavioral Therapy Workbook

Make the change!

Activity 1 – Setting up and Using a Journal

In chapter 4 for activity 1, you're asked to set up a journal. To journal, you need a notebook, or online document to record events from your days.

The most effective way to set up a journal is to make it as possible as possible.

In the Workbook…

It's suggested that at the very top of your journal page for each day, you should note down something you are thankful for today, so ensure you leave a prompt at the top of your diary – *Today, I'm thankful for…*

You then need to set up a table of four columns:
Event – So you can note down information about the event that triggered your reaction.
Feelings – How did this make you feel?
Actions – What did you do or how did you act in response to this event?
Thoughts – What thoughts did the event trigger?

You can note down positive and negative events in the table, but you should color-code these (black for negative and green for positive, for instance).

You should also leave a blank space at the end of your page too, so you can make a personal reflection in your journal.

Remember you need to use your journal every day for a number of weeks. You can assess your thoughts after one week and start to work on further CBT techniques, but you should keep on with your journaling and make it part of your daily routine.

On the next page is a journal sample document for you to copy and use and your own leisure.

Journal

Today, I am thankful for...

Events	Feelings	Actions	Thoughts

Personal Reflection

Activity 2 – Making Sense of it all

This activity is from chapter 4 and its aim is to help you make sense of your problems.

Take your journal, and highlight all of the negative thoughts, feelings and actions that you've identified so far.

Make a table:

Event	Feeling/Thought/Action	Cognitive Distortion	My ideal
Ran into someone at a party who used to bully me at school.	Felt angry, upset. Caused me to be snappy with others and leave the party early.	Blaming others.	Not to feel like I've done something wrong and should leave. I want to feel comfortable enough to stay and move on.

You need to note down the events from your journal in your table. You have to note down what you felt, thought and how you acted as a resulted. You then need to categorize the distortion, now above we use blaming others as our cognitive distortion in the example, now this doesn't mean that the bully is blameless.

Bullying is terrible, but for this exercise, if we think it's someone else's fault for the way we act/feel/think then we are blaming others. Maybe it is their fault and that's fine, but this process isn't about them, it's about you right now and how you can make a change. In the ideal part, simply make a comment on your ideal situation. *How did you want to act/feel/think?*

Once you've got them all down on paper and categorized, the fun can begin.

You'll find a blank copy of the above table for you to copy and use for your own leisure.
With this exercise, you start to realise just how your different events and problems affect you, and it really helps you get to the heard of the problem. Once we understand clearly why there is a problem, we are able to really consider what we must do, how and why.

The Making Sense of your Problems Table

Event	Feeling/Thought/Action	Cognitive Distortion	My ideal

Activity 3 – Why?

This activity is from chapter 5 of your CBT book.

Look closely at your cognitive distortions and using the boxes below, make some notes on the following questions as they will help you figure out why you feel the way you do;

What triggered the reaction exactly (something/one you seen, heard, a song perhaps)?

Why do you think you think you reacted in that way?

What's the worst that could happen if you faced this?

What would make the situation easier for you, or ease your worries?

Activity 4 – How to Identify your Bodily Reactions

This activity is from chapter 5 of your CBT book. It's so important to consider your bodily reactions, because sometimes it's not until we really consider this, that we realise what an affect our problems are having on our lives.

Follow the steps below:

1. Reflect back on your journal, and your work from activity 2.

2. Pick 2 or 3 key events that had the most distressing impact on you.

3. Note them down in the boxes below:

Event (what happened?)	How did my body react?

4. Think about this event and focus on how it made you feel, what it made you think and how you reacted. Now, think about how your body reacted and write this down. Did you keep thinking or reliving this event in your head? How long did the reaction last for (minutes, several days...)? Note down your responses.

5. Repeat step 4 for each key event you've noted down.

Sometimes our reactions last for 5-minutes, while others play on our minds and affect us for a number of days or weeks, so it's important to pinpoint this. Maybe it's still bothering you right now – if so, highlight this.

Activity 5 – Assessing and Challenging your Bodily Reactions

This activity is from chapter 5 and it's all about looking at those bodily reactions and making a judgement call. Throughout the course of this activity, you will need to reflect on what you know from activity 4.

*First of all, you need to A*nalyze*
Look for patterns and correlations between the way you think, feel and act, to the way your body has reacted. For example, if you were put in a stressful situation more than once, take yourself back to that day of the event and the days that follow and ask yourself the awkward questions:

How did my body react?	How does that correlate with the next event?
How was my appetite?	How did I sleep?
How was my mood/stress-levels?	Was I depressed/anxious?

Did I feel unwell/tired/unsocial on that day and the days that follow?	Is this normal for me?
How was I the day before this event?	When was I next/last happy?

Make some statements about your reactions to summarize your bodily reactions.

For example, every time I become anxious, I don't sleep and become unsocial, so I shut myself off from the world to regroup my thoughts. OR, every time I'm stressed out, I become moody and lose my appetite for 3 days.

***Challenge Yourself*itical*

You have started to recognize that your body reacts in a particular way to certain events. You can use this to your advantage by challenging and targeting your reactions.

If we use one of the examples from above:

Every time I become anxious, I don't sleep, and I become unsocial, so I shut myself off from the world to regroup my thoughts. There are four problems – the anxiousness, the lack of sleep, being unsocial, cutting ourselves off from the world. Why (and other problem questions) is always a good place to start. *Ask yourself why we feel or react in this way? What is it that we fear?*

By asking probing questions, we're challenging our reactions and although this may not remedy the immediate issues, being aware helps because we begin to understand why we react, feel and think in a particular way.

The ABC Model

The ABC model is referred to quite often in your CBT book, so here is the example of the model provided in your book in chapter 5.

	Irrational	*Rational*
A - Activating Event	Failed driving test	Failed driving test
B – Belief	Must pass the driving test on the first attempt.	<u>Would like</u> to have passed the driving test on the first attempt.
C - Consequence	Negative feelings of sadness, depression, anger, worthlessness.	Healthy feelings of sadness, and disappointment. Feeling of determination to pass next time.

Activity 6 – Using the ABC Model Yourself

This activity is in your CBT book from chapter 5. For this activity, you should make your own version of the table above and use some of the events from your journal and assess them, based on the ABC Model. 2-3 events will be sufficient to begin with, because for now, we're simply raising awareness of our beliefs rather than changing them.

Detail the activating event and then your beliefs on a rational and irrational level. Be honest with yourself when it comes to your irrational feeling. You will already be aware that this is irrational, but you can only challenge this in the future if this you are honest.

You then need to detail the consequences. *What are the consequences of your irrational thought? What are the consequences of your rational thoughts?*

*Repeat this sequence for some of the other events in your journal and then examine your responses in the table. *Can you see how our beliefs hold us back and stop us from moving forward?*

Using the ABC Model

Event 1	Irrational	Rational
A - Activating Event		
B – Belief		
C - Consequence		

Event 2	Irrational	Rational
A - Activating Event		
B – Belief		
C - Consequence		

Event 3	Irrational	Rational
A - Activating Event		
B – Belief		
C - Consequence		

Activity 7 – Self-Acceptance Exercise and Taking your own Advice

This activity is from chapter 6. It's important to be reflective in CBT, so look at your journal and reflect on one mistake you've made, or something about yourself that you don't like. This should be a something that really stands out for you and has instilled some fear. *You never want to experience that feeling, thought or action again!*

Imagine that a friend or family member feels like this or has made this mistake and they're distraught. What advice would you give them?

What mistake have I made?

What advice would I give if a family or friend made the same mistake? – Be as objective as possible.

Activity 8 – Exploring your Core Beliefs

This activity is from chapter 6 of your CBT book. This is a short activity

Activity 8 – Exploring your Core Beliefs
- Note down the situation that caused your initial problem and focus on how you felt or acted. What was the negative aspect?

  _____

- Really think about what this says about you. What do you think it suggests?

  _____

- Keep asking yourself why. Why did I feel like that? Why did I act like that?

  _____

- What do you think others will think about this?

  _____

- Why will they think that? Do you have any proof that people think this or is an assumption?

  _____

- What does this mean about the world or life?

  _____

- Why do you think the world will think or react like this? Again, what proof do you have of this?

  _____

- Look at your beliefs. Are there any common themes? For example, say your beliefs all point to a lack of self-belief, that's your theme. You then need to question why you have this self-belief and form your own probing questions based on your beliefs. When was the last time you really believed in yourself? What happened to make you stop believing in yourself?

  _____

Activity 9 – Plan your Exposure

This activity is from chapter 6 of your CBT book. Remember that exposure planning exposes you to situations or things that usually cause you to react in an irrational way, whether this be the way you think or act.

- Have a look in your journal from the last week, or your ABC Model and choose some regular events that set off your anxiety or cause some discomfort or distress. It must be something that you're willing to confront.

- Look at your notes and really think about how you feel and how you usually respond.

- Think about how you could respond in a rational and better way (how do you want to think, feel, act, next time this happens?).

- What does it suggest about your problems and your core beliefs?

- Make a plan to expose yourself to a situation or event that will spoke this feeling.

Make notes in the box below:

See the example below and then use the template on the next page for your exposure planning:

Triggering event	Exposure activity	Day/time of 1st exposure	Day/time of 2nd exposure	Outcome after 2nd exposure
What event triggers the feelings, thoughts and actions?	What happened last time? What will you do to avoid or cope with the situation? How?	Date and time of exposure activity.	Date and time of 2nd exposure activity.	How do you feel after the 2nd exposure? Did it get easier? How successful was it? What did you do differently?
Triggering event	Exposure activity	Day/time of 1st exposure	Day/time of 2nd exposure	Outcome after 2nd exposure

Activity 10 – Targeting Negative Belief Statements

We looked at this in chapter 6 of your CBT book. Do you remember the cereal brand example?
In this activity, we're going to challenge our core beliefs, once we work them out. If we go back to the driving test example, when we first looked at the ABC Model:
Belief: I must pass my driving test on my first attempt.

Based on this, our core belief is: *Failure is not an option.* There isn't a law that says we can't re-sit the driving test (or retake any test for that matter). This belief is false, it's irrational and it's unfounded. You need to respond to your core beliefs in a motivational way. Take a look at the example below:

Current Core Belief	Response to this belief
Failure is not an option	*I treat not winning or getting the results I want as a learning curve. Whenever I feel like I've failed or could've done better, I don't give up. I get back up, dust myself off, and feel more motivated than ever to do better next time.*

Think If a family or friend came to you with this belief, you wouldn't say *Sure, you're a failure, that's it for you now.* So, why do we do this to ourselves?
We are often our own biggest critic, when we should be a fan. We have the power to motivate ourselves and to make the change we crave.

Activity:

1. Make a table like the one above and make a list of your core values, assumptions and beliefs (there is a template for you to photocopy on the next page).

2. Get to the heart of your core belief and find out what it really means.

3. Make a positive statement in response to each of these.

4. Display these somewhere you can see them (post it notes on the wall, your notice board, or in the front of diary). You can refer to them whenever you have doubts.

Remember, we formed our belief system in the first place, so we can change it!

Current Core Belief	Response to this belief

Activity 11 – Relax and Reflect

This relaxation activity is in chapter 7 of your CBT book. You should approach this activity with an open mind. Read through the steps below before you begin.

- ✓ Find a relaxed position in either a sitting or laying position. Make sure you don't cross your arms and legs.
- ✓ Ensure you're somewhere quiet. It can be best if you are alone.
- ✓ Close your eyes and listen carefully.
- ✓ Breathe in for 5 seconds through the nose if possible. Hold for 1 second. Then breath out through the mouth for 5 seconds.
- ✓ Repeat the process around 10 times to regulate your breathing – you should be able to hear yourself breathe. Really concentrate.
- ✓ Your arms, legs and head should all feel relaxed and heavy.
- ✓ Fall into a natural breathing rhythm and focus on the breathing and how your chest rises and falls. Do this for a few minutes until you feel calm.
- ✓ When you're ready, open your eyes.
- ✓ Stay in the relaxed position but reflect back on the thing you were doing before the overwhelm kicked in. Give yourself some time to process this idea or thought again.
- ✓ If you start to feel overwhelmed again, return to the breathing technique – in for 5 seconds hold for 1 second, out for 5 seconds.

Make some notes about how you feel in the box below – when you come out of your relaxed breathing, what's the first thing you think about?

Activity 12 – Timed Muscle Relaxation

This activity is in chapter 7 of your CBT book. Time muscle relaxation can be great to help you relax and clear your mind. Read through the steps below and then give it a try. Remember to keep an open mind.

- ✓ Take yourself off to a quiet place, preferably somewhere you can lie down.

- ✓ Set your alarm for either 10 or 15 minutes.

- ✓ Tell yourself what time the alarm will sound – say it out loud and imagine the sound of your alarm in your head.

- ✓ Lay in a relaxed state. Don't cross any part of your body.

- ✓ Start breathing through your nose, in for 5 seconds, hold for 1 second, and out for 7 seconds.

- ✓ This will send a relaxing feeling through your body, allow it to flow from your shoulders, down, until it reaches your fingertips and then down your body to your toes.

- ✓ Your arms will feel heavy and you should continue to breathe, until you are in a fully relaxed state and then you can start to find your own breathing rhythm.

- ✓ Lay, in your relaxed state until your alarm sounds.

- ✓ You may wish to stay down for few minutes and refocus on your problems or issues, or you may just want to collect your thoughts.

- ✓ Take a couple of deep breaths before you sit up and ensure you move slowly, are your own pace.

Activity 13 – Your Ideal Life

This activity is from chapter 8 of your CBT book Before you begin reading, close your eyes and imagine your ideal life.

Focus on it. Visualize it!

How do you feel?

| |
| |

What changes would you need to make to get there?

| |
| |

What problems do you want to overcome?

| |
| |

What's your ideal?

| |
| |

You can use these probing questions to help you set your goals.

*Write down three things you want to focus on achieving – keep this for later.

Keep your vision in your mind!

Activity 14 – Work Towards your Ideal Life, with Positive Prediction Planning

Predict your future with positive prediction planning. This activity is from chapter 8 of your CBT book.

Look at the problems you've noted in your journal and complete the table below to create your five steps to success.

What's the problem?	What do you want?	Prediction Steps to Success
I'm stuck in a job I hate and it's making me feel stressed and depressed.	I want a job that I love and will enjoy.	1. Explore career opportunities 2. Upskill or train in appropriate areas. 3. Look for opportunities and apply for new jobs, that excite me. 4. Prepare for any interviews well and boss it. 5. Get a new job that I want!
		1. 2. 3. 4. 5

You should address at least three problems here from your journal, and you should reflect on your new core beliefs and your ideal, too!

The template for positive prediction planning is on the following page so you can copy the table and keep working on your problems. Working on your problems is an ongoing process, so this activity is something you can use over and over again.

What's the problem?	What do you want?	Prediction Steps to Success
		1. 2. 3. 4. 5
		1. 2. 3. 4. 5
		1. 2. 3. 4. 5

		1.
		2.
		3.
		4.
		5
		1.
		2.
		3.
		4.
		5

Activity 15 – Epiphany Moments

This activity is in chapter 8 of your CBT book. Follow the steps below and try to work out the epiphany moments in your life.

1. Think about some of the things you would like to change from your day. They could be something negative, but to keep in a positive mindset, we should think of these as our epiphany moments. We'll call these epiphany moments, because when you acknowledge your negatives and think about what you can change, or how they could've been better, it's a light bulb moment, or an epiphany.

2. You did some work earlier on your ideal life. Remember, this is what you are aiming for. This is now your main focus. Close your eyes and imagine the things you would like to change from the day. They are listed behind each other and they are forming a barrier, but your goal is within your grasp, *how can you overcome each barrier?* Leap over each barrier and grab your goal. *Great, you did it!*

3. Now, think of how you can prevent those events from occurring again by challenging your feelings, thoughts and behaviors, using your epiphany moments. Reflect

on each negative situation from your day, and imagine you handle it differently.

4. Close your eyes again and replay this out in your head but that you handle this in your ideal way. You're still reaching out for your goal and you're on target – you feel proud. Believe it!

5. Use positive phrases and say them out loud If 'this' ever happens again, this is how I will respond for a positive outcome.

Embedding how you want to react to something using positive phrases is a great way to stay positive and motivated about your future.

Activity 16 – Set your PAPER goals

Do you remember PAPER goals from your CBT book, in chapter 8? Based on your overall problems and beliefs so far, set 3-5 CBT goals using the PAPER framework, and 5 objectives or steps you need to take in order to reach your goal.

You can copy this template and use as you wish for future goal setting:

GOAL	STEPS/OBJECTIVES
1.	i) ii) iii) iv) v)
2.	i) ii) iii) iv) v)

3.	i)
	ii)
	iii)
	iv)
	v)
4.	i)
	ii)
	iii)
	iv)
	v)
5.	i)
	ii)
	iii)
	iv)
	v)

Activity 17 – Targeting your Triggers Technique

Activity 17 is from chapter 8. This activity is important as you need to be aware of, and feel able to target, your triggers.
In the activity, you should make a note of possible ways to target your triggers. If you find a pattern repeating itself, knowing how to target your trigger can prevent any episode of stress or anxiety.

Problem	Cause/Trigger	How can I target this?	Give yourself some encouragement
Note your problem or negative behavior here	*What are the causes or triggers?*	*Think about how you can target this issue. What's the solution?*	*Make a positive statement to encourage yourself – you got this!*

Activity 18 – Reflection Page

This activity is from chapter 9 of your CBT book. Reflection is extremely important because we should have time to consider the things that have happened in our lives.

First, think of two situations when you weren't assertive and note them in the table below.

Then think of how you could've responded or what you could've said to assert your own point of view, in an amicable and kind way. Often people mistake assertiveness as being forceful and sometimes even rude, but that's not the case. As assertive people, we tell others what we think in a nice way. In a way that respects their point of view but indicates our own perspectives. You have a right to have an opinion.

Event	How could I be more assertive?

Activity 19 – Being Aware

This activity is in chapter 9 of your CBT book. Just take a few minutes to note down some of your triggers and then answer the following questions:

1. Think about how you react when you are triggered – how do you feel, act and think?

2. What can you do to prevent your reaction?

3. Do you ever know in advance when you are going to be triggered, and can you do anything to stop it?

4. Is there anything you can do to avoid reacting in that particular way now that you're aware?

5. How do you think or wish you could respond when triggered in this way?

Activity 20 – Be Brave

We have to learn to be brave and face those uncomfortable things in life. It helps us grow! This activity is in chapter 10 of the CBT book.

There are four mindfulness techniques listed above: Breathing Exercises, Walking Meditation, Guided Meditation and Yoga Exercises.

Choose one of them, preferably a technique that you've never tried before (go on, be brave).

Try it as part of your daily routine for 1 week. Remember, now that you are more 'aware' you should be able to monitor this activity and its outcomes independently, so be objective, realistic and open minded.

Activity: *What did you do?*

Outcomes: *How did you feel? Did it have a positive/calming/motivational impact? Did you do anything that you wouldn't usually do? What could you do differently? How did it help?*

Monitor your progress – you can copy this table and use at your leisure:

Date/Day and time	Activity	Outcomes:

Activity 21 – Assess the Pros and Cons of hiring a Therapist

This activity is in chapter 11 of your CBT book. Now, we've established that it depends on the individual, whether or not a therapist is required but it's important that you make an informed decision. A great way to do this is to think about the benefits (pros) or drawbacks (cons)

Reflect on your own problems and beliefs with CBT in mind and map highlight the pros and cons of having a therapist. Make it personal to you!

Belief or Problem	Therapist Pros	Therapist Cons

Activity 22 – Reflect and Think

The reflect and think exercise is part of chapter 12. The idea is to reflect on your problems and beliefs and think about how or why they may need maintaining. Think about if they are long-term or short-term issues and what you will need to do to maintain them using CBT techniques.

Make notes below:

Activity 23 – Personal Maintenance Plan

The personal maintenance plan is part of chapter 12 of your CBT book. This is a really important part of CBT, because you've already practiced CBT, but you want to keep the momentum going. CBT isn't a magic formula, it's a way of life.

*Create a personal maintenance plan for yourself.

*Ensure you set at least three goals on the areas you want to improve or develop further with CBT.

*Think about how you will build the steps towards your goals, and your maintenance techniques into your routine.

You now know how to set effective goals, so it's time to set some new goals for the future.

Keep going – you got this!

GOALS:

1.

2.

3.

Steps for improvement/maintenance	How can I build them into my routine?

Reference List

[1] Albert Ellis Quotes. BrainyQuote.com, BrainyMedia Inc, 2019. https://www.brainyquote.com/quotes/albert_ellis_318498 accessed September 29, 2019.

[2] Mind. (2017). *Cognitive Behavioural Therapy (CBT)*. [online] Available at: https://www.mind.org.uk/information-support/drugs-and-treatments/cognitive-behavioural-therapy-cbt/#.XY6UCkZKjIU [Accessed 27 Sep. 2019].

[3] Dobson, K. (2010). *Handbook of cognitive-behavioral therapies*. 3rd ed. New York: The Guildford Press.

[4] McLeod, S. (2019). *Cognitive Behavioral Therapy*. [online] Simply Psychology. Available at: https://www.simplypsychology.org/cognitive-therapy.html [Accessed 27 Sep. 2019].

[5] Ellis, A. and Dryden, W. (1997). *The Practice of Rational Emotive Behavior Therapy*. 2nd ed. New York: Springer Pub. Co.

[6] McLeod, S. (2019). *Cognitive Behavioral Therapy*. [online] Simply Psychology. Available at: https://www.simplypsychology.org/cognitive-therapy.html Accessed 29 Sep. 2019].

[7] McLeod, S. (2019). *Cognitive Behavioral Therapy*. [online] Simply Psychology. Available at: https://www.simplypsychology.org/cognitive-therapy.html [Accessed 29 Sep. 2019].

[8] McLeod, S. (2019). *Cognitive Behavioral Therapy*. [online] Simply Psychology. Available at: https://www.simplypsychology.org/cognitive-therapy.html [Accessed 29 Sep. 2019].

[9] McLeod, S. (2019). *Cognitive Behavioral Therapy.* [online] Simply Psychology. Available at: https://www.simplypsychology.org/cognitive-therapy.html [Accessed 29 Sep. 2019].

[10] Klear Minds. (2015). *The History of Cognitive Behavioural Therapy (CBT).* [online] Available at: https://www.klearminds.com/blog/history-cognitive-behavioural-therapy-cbt/ [Accessed 29 Sep. 2019].

[11] Dobson, K. (2010). *Handbook of cognitive-behavioral therapies.* 3rd ed. New York: The Guildford Press.

[12] Klear Minds. (2015). *The History of Cognitive Behavioural Therapy (CBT).* [online] Available at: https://www.klearminds.com/blog/history-cognitive-behavioural-therapy-cbt/ [Accessed 29 Sep. 2019].

[13] NHS UK. (2019). *Cognitive Behavioural Therapy (CBT).* [online] Available at: https://www.nhs.uk/conditions/cognitive-behavioural-therapy-cbt/ [Accessed 27 Sep. 2019].

[14] Mind. (2019). *Cognitive Behavioural Therapy (CBT).* [online] Available at: https://www.mind.org.uk/information-support/drugs-and-treatments/cognitive-behavioural-therapy-cbt/#.XY6UCkZKjIU [Accessed Oct. 2017].

[15] Davro, B. (2019). *Best Picture Quotes and Saying Images about Peace of Mind - Quote Amo.* [online] Quote Amo. Available at: http://quoteamo.com/peace-of-mind-quotes/ [Accessed 27 Oct. 2019].

[16] Ackerman, C. (2019). *25 CBT Techniques and Worksheets for Cognitive Behavioral Therapy.* [online] PositivePsychology.com. Available at: https://positivepsychology.com/cbt-cognitive-behavioral-therapy-techniques-worksheets/ [Accessed 5 Oct. 2019].

[17] Edelman, S. (2006). *Change your thinking with CBT.* London: Vermilion.

[18] Macgill, M (2017) *What is depression and what can I do about it?* In Medical News Today. Available at: https://www.medicalnewstoday.com/kc/depression-causes-symptoms-treatments-8933 [accessed: 5, Oct, 2019]

[19] Effective Child Therapy. (2019). *Cognitive Behavioral Therapy - Effective Child Therapy.* [online] Available at: https://effectivechildtherapy.org/therapies/cognitive-behavioral-therapy/ [Accessed 5 Aug. 2015].

[20] Ackerman, C. (2019). *25 CBT Techniques and Worksheets for Cognitive Behavioral Therapy.* [online] PositivePsychology.com. Available at: https://positivepsychology.com/cbt-cognitive-behavioral-therapy-techniques-worksheets/ [Accessed 5 Oct. 2019].

[21] Ackerman, C. (2019). *25 CBT Techniques and Worksheets for Cognitive Behavioral Therapy.* [online] PositivePsychology.com. Available at: https://positivepsychology.com/cbt-cognitive-behavioral-therapy-techniques-worksheets/ [Accessed 5 Oct. 2019].

[22] Ackerman, C. (2019). *25 CBT Techniques and Worksheets for Cognitive Behavioral Therapy.* [online] PositivePsychology.com. Available at: https://positivepsychology.com/cbt-cognitive-behavioral-therapy-techniques-worksheets/ [Accessed 5 Oct. 2019].

[23] Ackerman, C. (2019). *25 CBT Techniques and Worksheets for Cognitive Behavioral Therapy.* [online] PositivePsychology.com. Available at: https://positivepsychology.com/cbt-cognitive-behavioral-therapy-techniques-worksheets/ [Accessed 5 Oct. 2019].

[24] Betterhealth.vic.gov.au. (2012). *10 tips for being assertive.* [online] Available at:

https://www.betterhealth.vic.gov.au/health/ten-tips/10-tips-for-being-assertive [Accessed 21 Oct. 2019].

[25] www.dictionary.com. (2019). *Definition of mindfulness | Dictionary.com*. [online] Available at: https://www.dictionary.com/browse/mindfulness?s=t [Accessed 22 Oct. 2019].

[26] Edelman, S. (2006). *Change your thinking with CBT*. London: Vermilion

[27] Psychology Today. (2019). *Mindfulness-Based Cognitive Therapy | Psychology Today*. [online] Available at: https://www.psychologytoday.com/us/therapy-types/mindfulness-based-cognitive-therapy [Accessed 22 Oct. 2019].

[28] Edelman, S. (2006). *Change your thinking with CBT*. London: Vermilion.

[29] Hayes, S. (2005). *ACT: Acceptance and Commitment Therapy*. [online] Getselfhelp.co.uk. Available at: https://www.getselfhelp.co.uk/act.htm [Accessed 22 Oct. 2019].

[30] Mind.org.uk. (2017). *Dialectical behaviour therapy (DBT) | Mind, the mental health charity - help for mental health problems*. [online] Available at: https://www.mind.org.uk/information-support/drugs-and-treatments/dialectical-behaviour-therapy-dbt/#.Xa9bxkZKjIU [Accessed 22 Oct. 2019].

[31] Caselli, G. (2019). *Metacognitive Therapy (MCT): An Interview with Prof. Adrian Wells*. [online] State of Mind. Available at: https://www.stateofmind.it/2012/05/adrian-wells-metacognitive-therapy/ [Accessed 22 Oct. 2019].

[32] Smith, D. (2018). [online] Brightlandhealth.com. Available at: https://www.brightlandhealth.com/single-

post/2018/07/31/Is-CBT-right-for-me [Accessed 21 Oct. 2019].

[33] Gray (2019). *The 1st CBT Session - What To Expect.* [online] Selfgrowth.com. Available at: https://www.selfgrowth.com/articles/the-1st-cbt-session-what-to-expect [Accessed 21 Oct. 2019].

[34] Branch, R. and Willson, R. (2012). *Cognitive Behavioural Therapy Workbook For Dummies, 2nd Edition.* Chichester: John Wiley & Sons.

www.ingramcontent.com/pod-product-compliance
Lightning Source LLC
Chambersburg PA
CBHW020253030426
42336CB00010B/743